MY LIFE AND MEDICINE

S. PADMAVATI

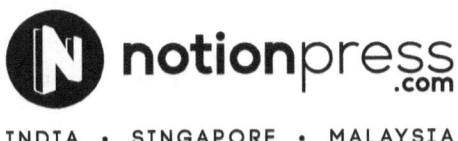

INDIA • SINGAPORE • MALAYSIA

Notion Press

Old No. 38, New No. 6
McNichols Road, Chetpet
Chennai - 600 031

First Published by Notion Press 2018
Copyright © S. Padmavati 2018
All Rights Reserved.

ISBN 978-1-64249-411-2

This book has been published with all reasonable efforts taken to make the material error-free after the consent of the author. No part of this book shall be used, reproduced in any manner whatsoever without written permission from the author, except in the case of brief quotations embodied in critical articles and reviews.

The Author of this book is solely responsible and liable for its content including but not limited to the views, representations, descriptions, statements, information, opinions and references ["Content"]. The Content of this book shall not constitute or be construed or deemed to reflect the opinion or expression of the Publisher or Editor. Neither the Publisher nor Editor endorse or approve the Content of this book or guarantee the reliability, accuracy or completeness of the Content published herein and do not make any representations or warranties of any kind, express or implied, including but not limited to the implied warranties of merchantability, fitness for a particular purpose. The Publisher and Editor shall not be liable whatsoever for any errors, omissions, whether such errors or omissions result from negligence, accident, or any other cause or claims for loss or damages of any kind, including without limitation, indirect or consequential loss or damage arising out of use, inability to use, or about the reliability, accuracy or sufficiency of the information contained in this book.

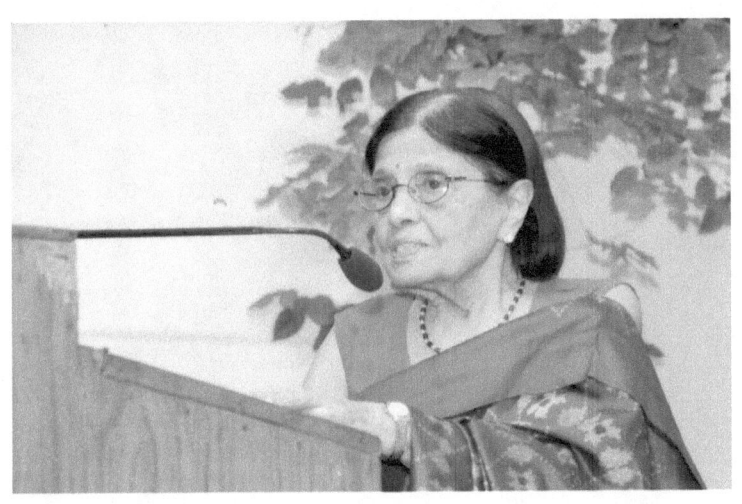

By
Dr. S. Padmavati
Padma Vibhushan, Padma Bhushan
MBBS (Rangoon), FRCP (London), FRCP (Edinburgh)
FAMS, FACC, FAHA, FESC
DSc (Hon.), PhD (Hon.)

Contents

Preface		*vii*
Chapter 1	My Early Years and Influences	1
Chapter 2	Early Education	15
Chapter 3	Postgraduate Education	25
Chapter 4	Professional Life	33
Chapter 5	Offshoots of Professional Life	53
Chapter 6	Historical Data and Ancient Systems of Medicine	77
Chapter 7	Heart Disease Today: Global Assessments	89
Chapter 8	Heart Disease in Neglected Groups	95
Chapter 9	Addressing Healthcare Delivery Gaps through Education	101
Chapter 10	Preventive Cardiology	107
Epilogue		*117*
Bibliography		*119*

Preface

Most budding young cardiologists today, faced with a dazzling array of gadgets and equipment, an even wider array of drugs and reports of spectacular cases of successful heart surgery, do not realize how recent all these are. Most doctors of my generation, born in the first decades of the Twentieth Century, have started from scratch and seen the specialty grow under their eyes. I am privileged to have witnessed the unfolding of the subject in my lifetime and contributed to some of it in India. Born in British Burma, and educated there and in the West, I was one of the few Indian women in this field, and had the privilege of knowing and working with some of the greatest cardiologists of the era.

This book contains memories and accounts of my own involvement in the field of heart disease. It also represents my philosophy with regard to Medicine and the subject of Cardiology. I shall be covering the development of cardiology in the last 50 years, the present situation worldwide—including that in India—and the role of preventive strategies. Scientific and technical developments have played a key role in advancing cardiology. As I will show, however, the greatest improvements in heart health are obtained by a combination of public health measures and lifestyle changes.

I shall also touch on my personal experiences with developments in the field during my tenure at Lady Hardinge Medical College, Maulana Azad Medical College, GB Pant Hospital, the All India Heart Foundation and National Heart Institute. My brush with Very Important Persons and Very Ordinary Persons as well as my Gurus will form part of the narrative. My personal areas of special interests, including research, preventive cardiology and international cardiology, along with awards and travels have also been outlined in the book.

Finally, I have provided a complete list of references which the reader may consult as required.

I would like to thank my parents and school teachers who taught me English and Mathematics, my nephew Dr. Inderjeet Mani and my former student Dr. Ratna Magotra for their the help with the script.

Chapter 1
My Early Years and Influences

I was born in 1919 in Magwe (also spelled Magway), a remote Upper Burma town situated on the banks of the Irrawaddy River. The birth took place in my parents' house, in the presence of a certified Burmese midwife. The fifth child of my parents, I had five siblings—an older brother, along with two other brothers and two sisters. Soon after my birth I was rolled in the mud for long life and good health because three other siblings had passed away soon after the birth of unknown causes. (This was done by an elderly aunt of my mother, who seems to have succeeded in her objectives).

Burma was then a province of British India (until its separation in 1937, when it was granted a degree of autonomy, while continuing as a colony). As India was several generations ahead of Burma in English-medium education, there were many Indians in the country who worked as doctors, lawyers, engineers and clerical staff. My father too belonged to this group, being a barrister.

Burma had a multi-ethnic population at that time. Besides the Burmese, there were many tribal peoples, Karens, Shans, Chins, Kachins, and Was. It had also quite a few Sino-Burmese, Anglo-Burmese, Anglo-Indians, Jews, Armenians, and Indian Muslims (Rohingyas) from what is now Bangladesh. The culture was very diverse, with influences from India as well as Nepal, Sri Lanka, Tibet, China, and Indonesia. All these different strains were reflected in day-to-day Burmese life. In those days, we all got along very well, with free entry into schools and technical institutions.

Magwe itself was in an oil-rich region of Burma, and continues to be so. We had Americans as well, working for the Burmah Shell oil company, and some would visit our home, as my father served as legal counsel to many of the oil barons. Overall, Burma was considered a land of milk and honey, where it was said *the land tickled with a hoe laughed with a harvest*. It was often contrasted with India and China which were both overpopulated, undernourished and in chronic poverty.

A Brief History of Burma

Like India, Burma is a land that has been settled for a long time. Traces of early settlements in Burma date as far back as 13,000 years. By 200 BC, the Tibeto-Burman Pyu people had created the first city-states. They adopted Theravada Buddhism, and their civilization lasted for nearly a thousand years. The Bamar people, who constitute the majority of Burmans today, entered the upper Irawaddy valley in the 9th Century. They went on to establish the Bagan Kingdom (1044–1287), and gradually the Bamar culture came to replace the Pyu states. There were many small kingdoms: Ava (1364–1555), Hanthawaddy Pegu (1287–1539), and the Shan states (1287–1563), until eventually the Konbaung Dynasty restored the kingdom and ruled from 1752–1885.

Meanwhile, in Lower Burma, the Mon people were the majority, having already established the Buddhist Dvaravati and Haripunchai kingdoms in Thailand by the Seventh Century. However, in Burma, they had come under Bamar rule by the Eleventh Century. The British arrived relatively recently, establishing colonial rule in Upper Burma only in 1825 and Lower Burma in 1885, when the last Burmese king Thibaw was escorted away from the Mandalay Palace in a bullock cart and exiled to Ratnagiri on the west coast of India, where he died thirty one years later.

The Japanese occupied Burma in 1942, remaining there until the Second World War ended in 1945. After that, the country returned to British hands, while negotiations for independence began. In 1947, Burma became independent. Soon after, the entire cabinet led by General Aung San was assassinated. Chaos followed, with the country undergoing five decades of military rule from 1962–2015, when a civilian government took over with the key portfolios still with the military.

Indians had been coming to Burma for a long time, but their numbers swelled under British rule. Their dominant presence in the British administration made them a target for Burmese nationalists. In 1930, Indian workers at the port of Rangoon (now called Yangon) went on strike and were replaced temporarily by Burmese workers. When the strike ended, clashes between the two groups led to riots, with over two hundred Indians killed, with the riots soon spreading across the country. Later, during the Depression of the 1930's, moneylenders from the Chettiar community in South India began to foreclose on Burmese rice farmers, leading to further animosity on the part of the Burmese. Many of the Indians, including myself along with the other women in the family, fled at the start of the Japanese occupation in 1942. When Burma achieved independence, the Indians still residing there were not granted citizenship, which was restricted to those who arrived before 1823. In 1964, with the military's nationalization of private industry, 300,000 Indians lost their property and were forced to leave the country.

Grandparents

My paternal grandfather was a landowner in Gobichettipalayam, near Coimbatore, Tamil Nadu. He died at an early age, leaving my grandmother a young widow with twelve children, six boys and six girls, to bring up. The family had inherited land from the time before 1800, and it was passed on from generation to generation. However, there were now in debt from the lands. The boys were educated in Bangalore in the house of my paternal grandmother's brother and the girls were educated up to the fourth standard.

My paternal grandmother had received no formal education and could only sign her name in Tamil. Widowed at an early age, she raised all her children single-handed. She sent the boys for higher education to Bangalore and Madras, while the girls were married off around the ages of twelve and thirteen. She accomplished all this while also endowing, in Gobi, a primary girls' school and a shrine to Lord Ganesha. The shrine is popular even today, and members of the family visit it whenever they go to Gobi. In spite of her lack of education, my grandmother went to court several times over land disputes, many of which she won. In these disputes, she took on the the male-run village council, breaking with centuries of tradition. I guess she was one of my earliest female role models! Her legal activities were also influential in guiding her favourite son, my father, to seek greener pastures abroad through the profession of law. Through the money he earned, he helped to pay off the debts and gave financial assistance to his brothers, nieces and nephews whenever required.

My maternal grandparents were orthodox Brahmins from Komaralingam, southeast of Coimbatore. They were steeped in the traditions of ancient texts and Carnatic music. My maternal grandmother had six sons and two daughters, who were brought up as traditional Brahmin children. The boys were all graduates and knew English well, while the girls were married off at the age of eleven or twelve after studying English up to the fourth standard. Both girls were well-educated in Carnatic music.

Parents

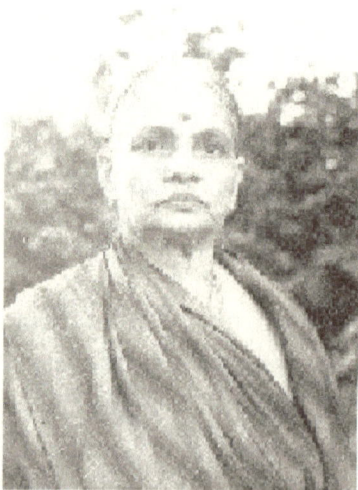
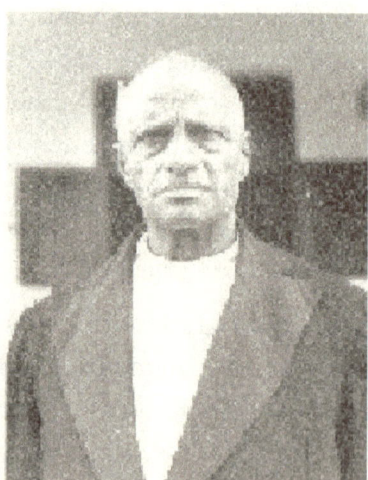

My father trained as a lawyer, acquiring his BA and BL degrees in Bangalore. He subsequently came to Burma and settled in practice in Magwe, the district headquarters. During his stay, he travelled frequently to Rangoon, where the Supreme Court is located now. He went to London for a while and was called to the Bar at Lincoln's Inn in 1913.

Even though my father was not at all superstitious by nature, he had to undergo purification ceremonies on his return because in those days, it was considered a sin to cross the seas. Women in his family were unable to find suitable matches for marriage because he had gone abroad. This seems unbelievable today, when migration to foreign countries is almost the norm and the goal of many young people.

My father was very fond of books of all types, a trait which his children inherited. Among his favourites were the accounts of the Chinese travellers Fa Hien (now spelled Faxian) and Hiuen Tsang (now Xuanzang). He was very fond of spending time outdoors and embarking on long walks, and never missed going out in the evenings, no matter how late it became. He was also an expert swimmer. I remember many joyful hours with my siblings and him, splashing around in the Irrawaddy River. My father never scolded his children, so much so that my mother said that it was no use complaining to him about our misdeeds, which were many. He was very helpful and respectful to everyone, irrespective of caste or creed. He was awarded the title of Rai Bahadur by the British and became President of the Magwe Municipality.

My father was never inclined towards superstition and always tried to understand the rationale behind every action. He often questioned the Hindu pundits about the scriptures and Sanskrit *shlokas* as they were blindly repeating the verses and did not understand what these meant. He was also very much ahead of his time in encouraging the education of women, instead of following the backward customs of his forefathers, who preferred that girls study only until the fourth standard. Consequently, he was vehemently opposed to having daughters married off early. He was also deeply involved in all our studies, especially those of my sisters and I. It is thanks to his influence on my education that I am where I am today.

My father's life changed drastically once the Japanese invaded Burma in 1942. While my mother, sisters, my eldest brother and I fled on the last plane out, my father remained behind with two other brothers, hoping to take care of his property in Magwe and Rangoon, along with what remained of his practice. None of that came to pass. Instead, he was interned, and his fate was unknown until after the war. Eventually, when my father rejoined us at home in India, his health was not that good, but he lived happily for another decade in Coimbatore, dying on Christmas Eve in 1954.

My mother was born in 1899, the sixth child in her family and the first girl. As a result, she was pampered by everyone. As was the custom in those days, she was married at the age of eleven. However, she did not join my father until much later. Even after her marriage, my grandmother would treat her like the child she was. My maternal uncles were close to us, and were graduates, well-versed in English. Two of them even went on to be Deputy Collectors, which was a very high post in those days. When my mother turned nineteen, two of her brothers escorted her to Burma, by which time my father was well settled in his practice there. Their knowledge of English helped them to secure excellent jobs.

I remember my mother as a very beautiful lady, remaining so well into her old age. Her complexion was the envy of everyone who knew her. She never used any cosmetics. An oil bath twice a week and sparing use of soap, coupled with the use of powdered *dals* with aromatics, were part of her usual regimen. Today, people pay large sums of money for such treatment in spas and beauty parlours. My siblings and I too used to have oil baths, but only once a week, because we had to go to school.

My mother was a home-maker and an excellent cook specializing in south Indian food, often making delectable snacks and sweets for us. She always had plenty of domestic help, but she nevertheless did all the cooking until about 1937. She was also devoted to her children. She was well versed in Sanskrit and taught Tamil to all of us at home. The only reason we never read any Tamil literature or Sanskrit books was because they were unavailable in Burma. However, my mother would narrate stories from religious texts, and we knew all about them from a young age.

My mother was broad-minded and did not discriminate against people who practiced Christianity or Islam. She had a statue of Buddha in her shrine and used to feed Burmese monks when they came for alms. She would work tirelessly throughout the day and only indulge in half an hour of rest in the afternoons, after which she would resume activities like sewing clothes for us children or quietly reading books written in Tamil or Sanskrit. I remember that she used to get from Rangoon a Tamil weekly, the *Ananda Vikatan*, and a newspaper the *Swadeshi Mitran*, from Rangoon. My father used to subscribe to *Modern Review* and *Indian Review*, which gave all the news of importance from India.

Siblings

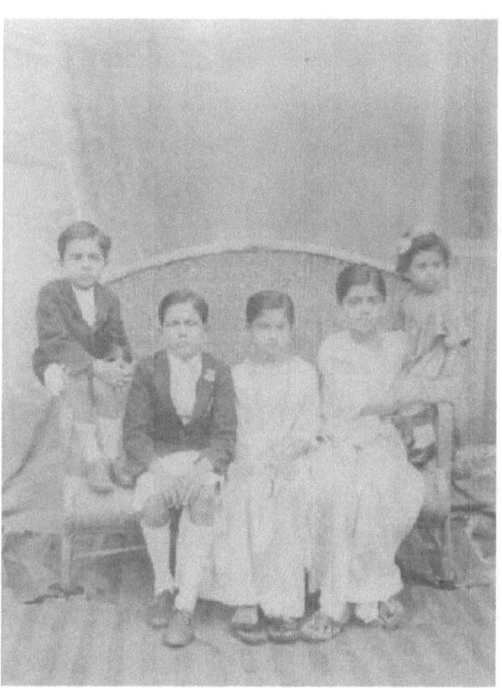

I had five siblings, three brothers and two sisters. My eldest brother Chellana, who was about 10 years my senior, was born in India with an infantile hemiplegia on the right side, which grew worse with age. In spite of this he went on to obtain his B.A. in Philosophy, with Honours, from Judson college at Rangoon University and later went to London and obtained an LLB after which he was also called to the bar. A brilliant and well-read bachelor, due to his disability my father felt it was advisable for him to leave with the women on the last flight out of Burma, in 1942. Chellana settled in Coimbatore, and died in 1975.

My other two brothers were engineers. Ramu, the elder one, joined the Burma Railways, and remained behind working under the Japanese when we left. He went to the USA after the war ended and studied at Harvard University and the University of Illinois. He settled there, marrying an American woman of Swedish descent, and had three children there. One is a doctor, another a mathematics teacher, and the third is a biologist. Ramu passed away there in 2011.

During the war, my younger brother Kittu learnt Japanese and became an interpreter for the Kempetai (the Japanese secret service). He was able to shift my father to safer places, thanks to information he received from the Kempetai. After the war, he trained in the UK on Opencast Coal mining and following long service in India retired as a superintending engineer, returning to the family house in Coimbatore. He had two children, a business executive and a professor, both settled in the USA. He passed away there in 2015.

My sister Saraswathi was four years younger and was educated in Queen Mary's College, Madras. She was very good at sports and had a flair for languages, including Burmese. She received an M.A. in education and worked for a while as a teacher. She took over responsibilities as a full-time homemaker when she married Foreign Service Officer P.R.S. Mani, a distinguished former war correspondent who retired as Ambassador of India to Sweden. She travelled with her husband to all his diplomatic postings around the world. After her husband retired, they settled in Bangalore. She had two boys, educated at a boarding school in India, and they would come down to visit me during their summer vacations. One is a doctor, settled in the USA, and the other is a computer expert, who after a career in the USA, became a writer and settled in Thailand. Their mother passed away in 1995 of cancer. Her husband remained in Bangalore after her death, until he too passed away, in 2011.

My youngest sister Janaki was a neurologist with an FRCP from London and Edinburgh. She was a very bright student and was also very fond of swimming. She was also a pioneer in neurology in India. She started working at the prestigious Christian Medical College, Vellore and later moved to Delhi to Safdarjung Hospital and subsequently to G.B. Pant Hospital. She became Head of the Neurology Department twice at G.B. Pant Hospital. She carried out a substantial amount of research and travelled a great deal. She moved in with me in 1985 after she retired. She continued to practice until she was disabled, but remained an Honorary Consultant at the National Heart Institute. She passed away in 2010. There is a lecture in her name at the National Academy of Medical Sciences given every year.

Now, my family has expanded, with four nephews, three nieces, and three grand-nephews and three grand-nieces, most of them living in the USA. They visit frequently, and we are very fond of one another.

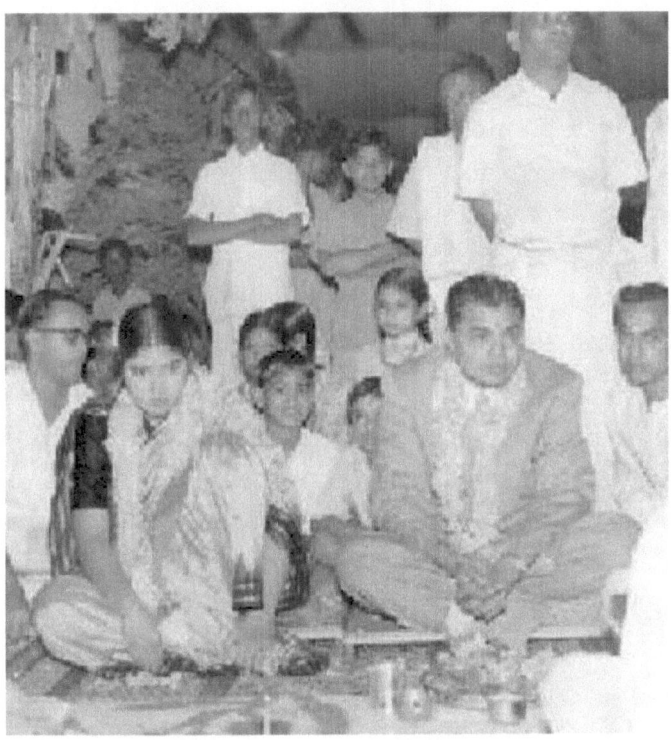

Younger Brother's Marriage

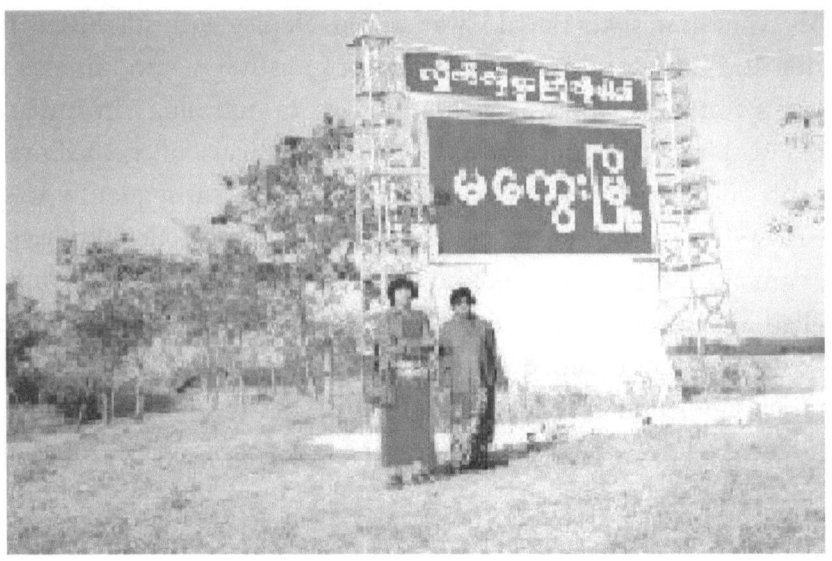

Sign Board at Magwe

Family Life

Our house in Magwe is, as far as I know, still standing. We had a one-acre compound with a tennis court, and quarters for my father's clerks and the domestic help. We also had a cowshed big enough for three cows. As Indians, we were used to a diet in which milk and dairy products were an integral part. However, milk was not easily available in Burma as the locals use only condensed milk for their coffee, tea being drunk without milk and sugar. Our cows provided all the milk for our daily consumption.

The house had two parts, the larger one containing living quarters, my father's office, and our living rooms and bedrooms. The other was a smaller house, referred to as our Mother's house, with the kitchen, *puja* room, dining room and bathrooms. We had no electricity or running water until 1937. The servants used to draw water from a well, which was still functional in 2000, when I last visited it. The well was next to the bathrooms, and the servants used to draw all the water for our baths from the well and pour them into dispensing vessels. They were two big banyan trees next to the well, which must have seen a lot of history, as they were still standing in 2000.

My oldest brother Chellana was not in Magwe most of the time. He was taken to Maymyo by my uncle for schooling as there were no schools in Magwe. He used to come only during the holidays. My youngest sister Janaki was the pet of the family. As she was my junior by nearly a decade, she was educated in Magwe and finished her school in Rangoon, as by that time we had all moved to Rangoon for college.

We children enjoyed each other's company immensely. My brother Ramu was very naughty and gave my mother no end of problems. He used to stand on the parapet of the top floor and threaten to jump if his wishes were not agreed to. We used to dodge our mother as much as possible. I like to look back on those childhood days in Magwe as a very pleasurable time.

In terms of sports, we used to play tennis together in our courts, go swimming and overall had a great time. We used to play chess with our mother. She had a great skill at the game and used to beat us all the time. We also played cards with our mother and amongst ourselves. Badminton was a sport we enjoyed with our Burmese friends.

As children, we would be given a monthly dose of castor oil, which was considered absolutely mandatory for children as a cure for all diseases. Being a purgative, castor oil was something we dreaded and despised, and I remember my mother chasing us with the castor oil bottle. My siblings and I also all came down with chicken pox together and were kept in a separate room with *neem* leaves thrown at us from time to time by our mother, as *neem* was considered a cure for the disease. Our chicken pox seemed more or less painless except for the disfigurement.

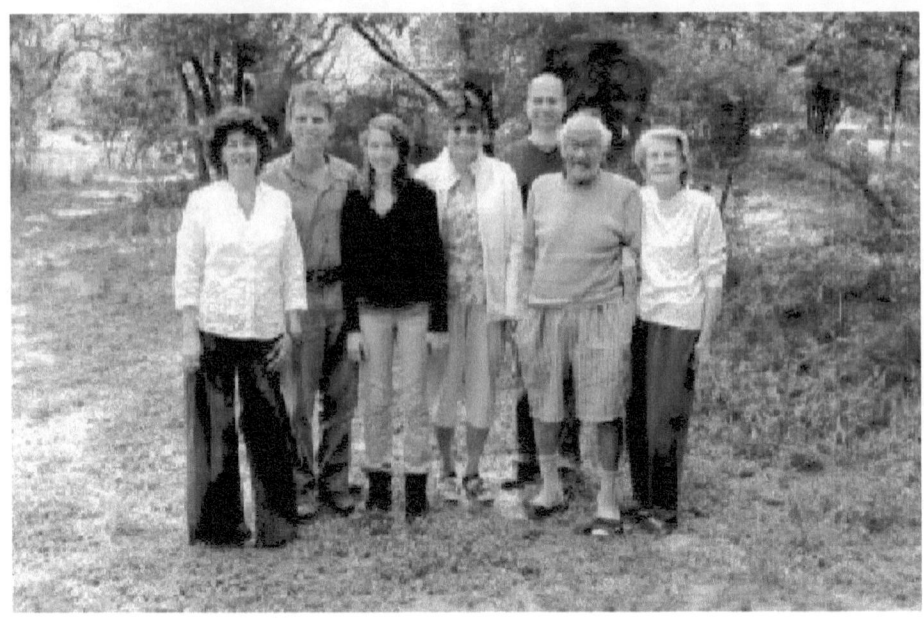

My brother in USA with his Family

Like our father, my siblings and I were all fond of reading. While in our teens, we read the classics, with Shakespeare being our favourite. We also eagerly devoured the words of the Brontës, Arthur Conan Doyle, P. G. Wodehouse and George Bernard Shaw, among others. My interest in French, Swedish and German authors (in translation) developed around the same time. Reading such a wide range of authors and their works helped me and my siblings to formulate a diverse world view and learn a great deal that came in useful in later life.

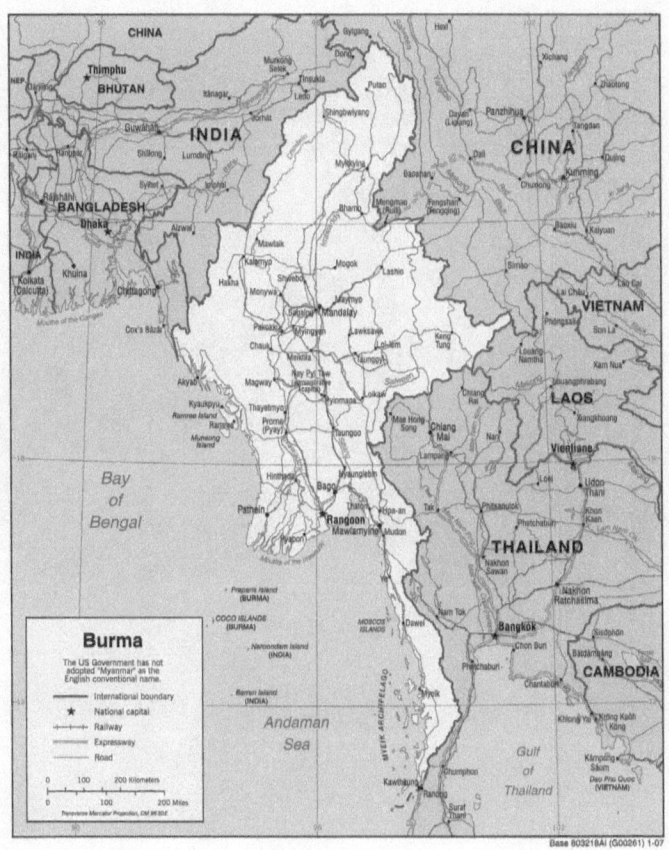

Map of Burma

My mother also taught us Carnatic music, which she would teach many girls of the south Indian community in Magwe. The multi-talented woman that my mother was, she also taught herself to play the violin. We were given lessons in harmonium, violin and piano. My love for Carnatic music was thus nurtured, and I later also developed a strong liking for western classical music. I am glad to have had all these influences while growing up.

Overall, ours was a happy childhood. Our parents taught us to value a simple life focusing on academic pursuits and sports, and we were well-adjusted to Burma.

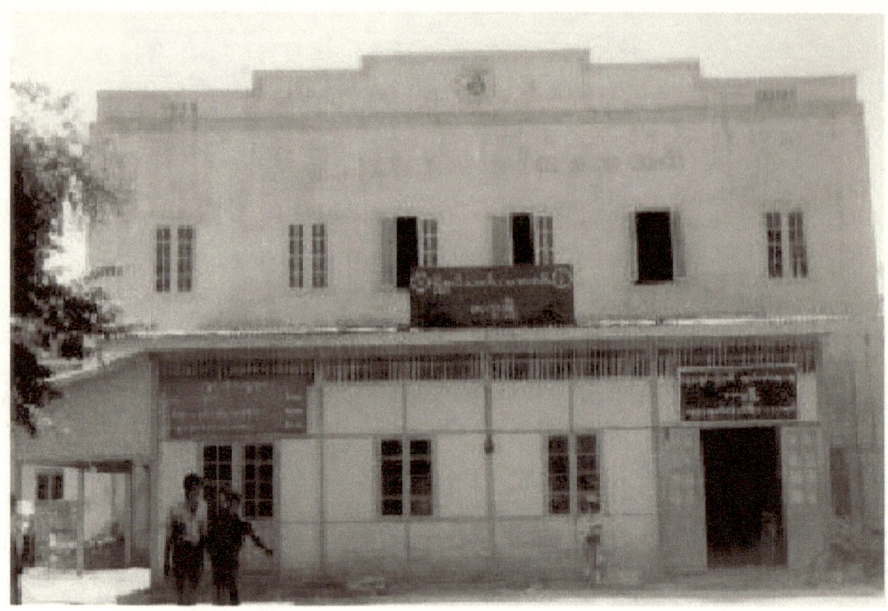

Magwe House

Chapter 2
Early Education

Magwe

Ours was a highly polyglot household, and we got used to the habit of switching between multiple languages. As children, we used to speak in Tamil to our mother, in English to our father, in Hindustani to our domestic help who were from UP and Bihar (and illiterate), and in Burmese among ourselves. As a child, I initially went to a Burmese school before English-medium schools were opened. To this day I can read, write and speak the language fluently. In later life, long after we left Burma, my siblings and I still spoke to each other in Burmese.

While the Hindustani we spoke to the servants in those days was a mix of Hindi and Urdu, we also learned Hindi and Urdu separately from a tutor, Mr. Ghosh. He would come home to teach us as there was no school for these languages in Magwe. However, the influence of the servants' Hindustani was stronger, so I speak that rather than proper Hindi. I found Urdu more akin to Hindustani, and it came in handy when I visited Pakistan in 1989. (In later life, I also had to study French and German from private tutors in England while studying for the MRCP, as one could score higher marks if one knew these languages.)

When I graduated from my English-medium high school in Magwe, I stood first in the province and won many prizes, distinctions and gold medals, which was unprecedented for a girl. As a result, the school received huge grants and a new building. My teachers were mostly Indians or Anglo-Burmese, along with a few Burmese. I would like to pay tribute to my teachers who taught me English literature and Mathematics. Their lessons and my interactions with them have shaped my life a great deal.

I got interested in medicine when I came into contact with the Licensed Medical Practitioners (LMPs) who were working in the district hospital in Magwe. These doctors worked under civil surgeons, who visited the hospitals from time to time. The LMPs were my first inspiration for choosing the medical profession. They were the fount of all knowledge, and I found that they were very pleasant and extremely approachable. Unfortunately, this cadre was abolished by the British and later by the Indian government. Apart from being extremely impressed by these doctors, I also chose medicine because career options for women were limited in those days.

University Education in Rangoon

After high school, I joined Rangoon University, where one had to take the intermediate exam and enrol in order to subsequently study medicine. Founded in 1929, the university was modelled after the British university system of the time. The director of the Rangoon University was one Dr. Schloss, who was a British Jew. The British headed all the departments except for Burmese and Pali. It was the Indians who formed the second-largest group. There were very few Burmese on the staff. This was because English-medium education was not common in Burma at that time. The head of the English department was Mr. B.R. Pearn, whom I found to be a very good teacher. Dr. Quayle headed the physics department, while Dr. Peacock was the head of chemistry and Dr. F. J. Meggitt the head of biology.

After my intermediate studies at Rangoon University, I was admitted to Rangoon Medical College (RMC). I stayed at Inya Hall—the women's hostel throughout my time at college. Though it was about 10 kilometres from the Medical College and Rangoon General Hospital, there was an efficient bus system that was easily accessible. I used to leave at 7 am and return after 6 pm on most days. The hostel was modern, with single and double rooms, tennis and squash courts, and a swimming pool within easy reach.

Founded in 1929, RMC was staffed entirely by Indian Medical Services doctors, who were all British ex-army men and worked as heads of departments. The second in line were all Indians, who had acquired degrees in India. All of the staff were extremely well disciplined and good at their work, and the students enjoyed their studies, as each class had no more than fifty people. The nurses were all mostly Karen. Only a small number of staff were Burmans, due to the fact that teaching was in English.

The medical college trained MBBS students (enrolled in a five-year course) and LMP students (enrolled in a three-year course). I think this was a very good arrangement as the same equipment and staff were used to train students of both programs. As I recall, the head of the RMC was Col. J.C. Barrat, who was also a professor of anatomy. The head of physiology was Col. C.F.J. Cropper, the head of bacteriology and pathology was Col. Malone, and the head of ophthalmology was Col. Maccormack. Col. R.V. Morrison headed the department of medicine, while Col. McDonald looked after the department of surgery and Col. Treston the department of obstetrics and gynaecology. The rest of the staff were Indians.

At the RMC, the cases one saw were very different from what one sees today. I saw mostly infections such as diarrhoea, dysentery (this was before the use of antibiotics), pulmonary tuberculosis, pneumonia, and typhoid. I also encountered diseases of nutritional deficiency such as rickets, osteomalacia, beri beri, diabetes and epidemic dropsy. We also came across patients with tetanus and rabies at the Infectious Diseases Hospital. We did not see any of the chronic diseases which dominate patients at general hospitals today. The anti-bacterial drug Prontosil was introduced around 1938 and hailed as a wonder drug. Sulfa drugs were the only anti-bacterial prescription of the time.

My friends in the hostel were mostly of my age group and a few seniors. We all got along very well. The warden was Anglo-Indian, and the assistant warden Burmese. We had to dine with the warden once a week at the central table. The food was all non-vegetarian, and I used to obtain vegetarian food from one of the professors at the university. I also sought out vegetarian food from neighbouring food stalls like many of the other girls. However, I must admit that I have tasted every kind of meat such as beef, pork, mutton, chicken, fish and prawns. This was because I had many non-vegetarian friends who were Anglo-Indian, Burmese, Anglo-Burmese, Jews and Armenians. They used to call me a 'grass eater' and made me taste all these foods!

As I was fond of sports, which my father had encouraged all along, I played tennis, table-tennis, and squash, and swam a lot as these sporting facilities were available close by. I managed to win prizes in swimming and tennis. Many of my friends in the hostel have passed away, but some including the sportspersons are alive today.

Apart from medicine, my other interests in college included reading and listening to music, especially Carnatic and western classical. My reading choices tended towards inspirational biographies and English literature, both classics as well as contemporary writing. Astronomy was also one of my interests, and I never forget to watch eclipses, all thanks to an uncle of mine, who was very interested in Astronomy without relying on the use of a telescope. I have also long been fascinated by animals and birds. I have had three dogs as pets but when they died, my heart broke and I did not adopt any more. I have kept up the hobbies of reading and birdwatching till today. My favourite bird is the striped woodpecker, but it is less seen today because of competition from bigger birds.

I passed my MBBS examinations in 1941 in the first division with distinction in Anatomy, Physiology, Pathology, Forensic Medicine, Hygiene and Public Health. I was ranked the best outgoing student. Amongst those who passed out with me were two Anglo-Burmese, two Muslims (one Bangladeshi and one Iranian), three Indians, including myself. Three were women and the rest were men. There were no Burmese in my class. I also completed internships in Rangoon General Hospital and Dufferin Hospital.

Relocation to India

While I was obviously pleased with my results, my whole world was suddenly turned upside down when the Japanese attacked Pearl Harbor in Hawaii on December 7, 1941.

A week later, the Japanese began attacking Burma. On the morning of December 23, three Japanese air squadrons attacked the airport at Rangoon, which was then also the British Royal Air Force (RAF) base. Then two more squadrons attacked the city centre, with more than a hundred Japanese planes altogether. There were fierce air battles involving RAF fighter planes as well as the American Flying Tigers defending against the Japanese, which led to many aircraft on both sides being shot out of the sky. However, the Japanese were able to inflict maximum damage to both the airport and the Rangoon city centre. Most of the wooden buildings were flattened, with many people charred to a crisp. There was absolute chaos everywhere, and my ears were full of the sounds of bombs and gunfire! As people fled their collapsing houses and shops, there were stampedes, and many people died as a result of being trampled. Altogether nearly 2,000 civilians were estimated killed.

I had to leave Rangoon for Magwe immediately. My father was ordered by the British government to vacate his house within 48 hours of the war being declared. The following month, in January 1942, the Japanese Army crossed over from Thailand into southern Burma. They soon captured Moulmein, in the Salween River Delta, after routing the 17th Indian Infantry Division. On March 7, lacking reinforcements to defend Rangoon, whose port and oil refinery had already been destroyed by the Japanese, the British commander-in-chief General Harold Alexander ordered the city to be evacuated. Prisoners in jail were released, and the Rangoon Zoo left open.

This zoo was a particularly excellent one and I had very fond memories of visiting it! The writer Amitav Ghosh, in his riveting blog on the events of the time, quotes Leslie Glass, a British civil servant posted there: "One afternoon, I joined in a bizarre and melancholy foray to shoot all dangerous animals in the zoo, as all their keepers had decamped. Tigers, panthers and poisonous snakes were killed and the deers released in the park, except for one which we shot for fresh meat. When we had gutted the poor beast, we threw its entrails into the lake and great fish thrashed and swirled in the course of their unusual meal."

To add to the sense of gathering disaster, the Indians in Rangoon decided to flee. Since they made up much of the working-class of the city, that crippled the city further. The docks were abandoned, leaving supply-laden ships in the port to be bombed to smithereens. Ghosh speculates that the Indians may have been worried about their future in case the Japanese were victorious, and they also may have feared the Burmese mob, given that the violence meted out towards Indians in the 1930s (mentioned earlier) was not long past. By April 16, the Japanese had captured Magwe, and by May 1, Mandalay. The Burma Corps, that is, the British Indian Army in Burma, were forced to beat a hasty retreat all the way back to Imphal in Manipur, India, traveling by road and track among the sick, wounded and starving refugees.

As they retreated north, the British followed a Scorched Earth policy, destroying anything that might be of use to the enemy, including bridges, railways, irrigation, oil refineries, and farms. The oilfields near Magwe were set on fire. This Scorched Earth policy has been criticized a lot. While beating their retreat, there was hardly any resistance offered, such as anti-aircraft defences, or substantial army resistance. The war was the price the country paid for separation from India in 1937. Because they had no ally in India, the Burmese themselves hardly had any soldiers.

From Magwe, my mother, sisters, my disabled brother and I flew out on the last plane in March 1942, with Japanese bombers already attacking the airport shortly before. The men—my father and the two other brothers—were left behind and we did not know anything about their fate, in spite of the efforts of the Red Cross. Our only connection to that part of the world was through radio, which we would listen to eagerly everyday.

We came via Chittagong and Kolkata to Tamil Nadu and settled in Coimbatore, which was my parents' hometown. All of us were warmly received by relatives from both my father's and mother's side. Although we had lost all our property and assets in Burma, we managed to soon buy a house, close to where my mother's family lived. The house was used by members of the family until 2015, when it was sold to a developer.

During my years in India, I did not find anything much to do. I joined several Indian Hospitals for short periods. After the war ended in 1945, I joined the Civil Affairs Service (Burma), or CAS (B), set up in India to help with the reconstruction of Burma. I worked with other exiles from Burma and finally managed to revisit Burma. Once there, I was able to travel with another army doctor by truck and bullock cart through a war-ravaged landscape, eventually tracking my father and my younger brother down. It is hard to forget, after all these years, the intense emotions that we three experienced when we were at last reunited! It had been almost four years of separation, without our knowing if they were still alive!!

From there, in 1946, I went to the U.K. as a Burma state scholar.

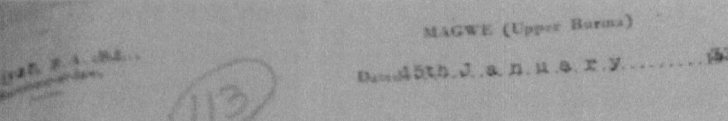

Letter From My Father While I Was in College

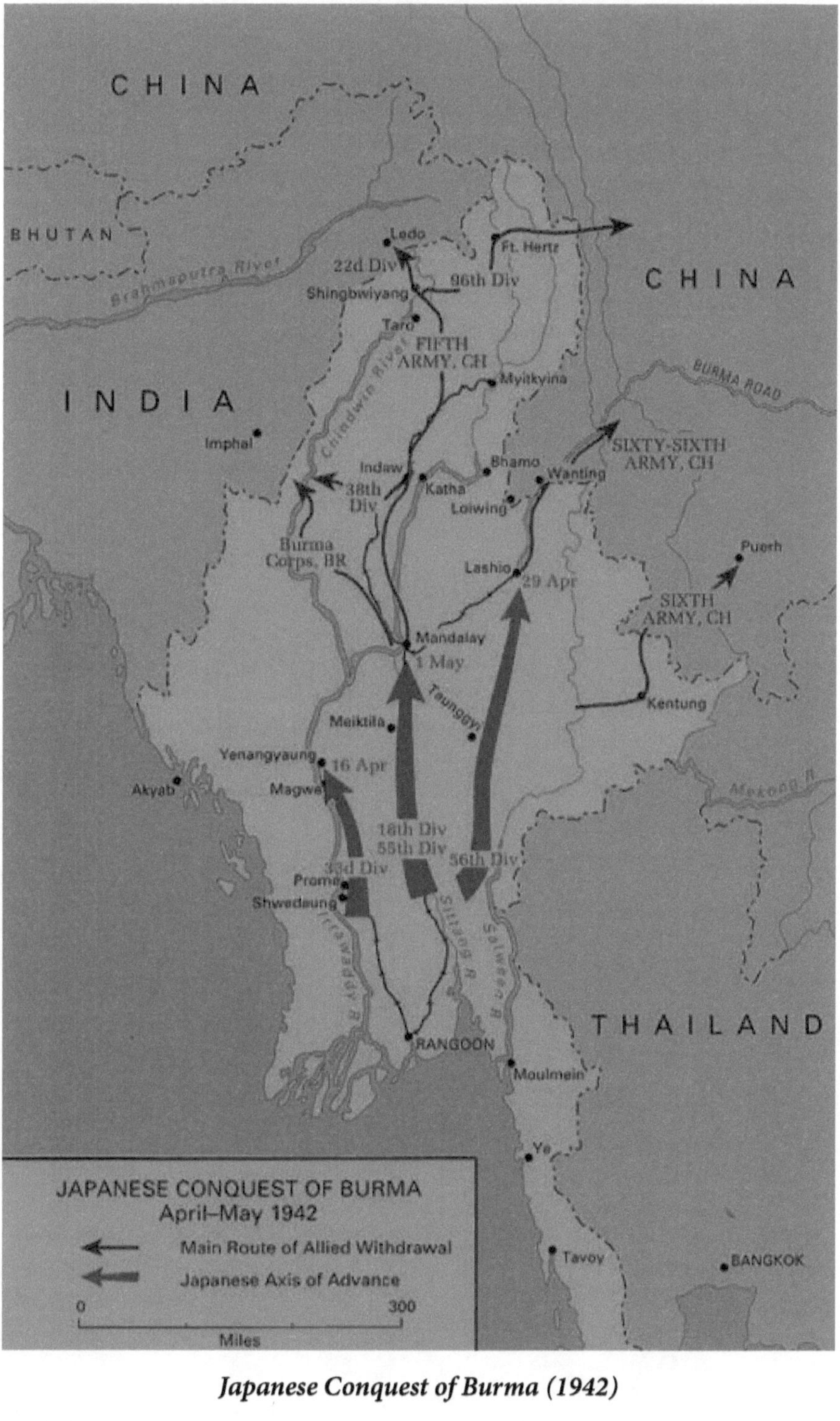

Japanese Conquest of Burma (1942)

Chapter 3
Postgraduate Education

Doctors today are better off than those of earlier generations, but modern medical equipment has resulted in the diminishing of their clinical acumen. They have become too dependent on pathological tests and monitoring devices, and intuitive diagnosis is rare these days. While technological advancements are advantageous, we cannot overlook the nurturing of clinical acumen. I was fortunate to have the benefit of post-graduate studies in different phases and in different countries. This variety of experience is what made me aware of the different approaches to cardiology across the globe early in my career.

United Kingdom

I went to the UK in 1946 for post-graduate studies with an MRCP in mind, as it was considered the ultimate medical qualification in those days. I was posted to the National Heart Hospital, London as part of my training. This hospital was founded in 1857, where it was known as the Hospital for Diseases of the Heart, and was the first hospital in the world dedicated to the study and treatment of heart disease. (The first heart transplant in the UK took place there in the 1960's, as well as the first successful coronary angioplasty and coronary stent implantation in the UK.) At the National Heart Hospital, the superb clinical acumen of giants of the time, Sir John Parkinson, Evan Bedford and Paul Wood could not but impress and inspire.

Parkinson (1885–1976) is widely regarded as the founder of modern British cardiology. He is well-known (with Paul White and Louis Wolff) for the definitive description of what is now known as Wolff-Parkinson-White syndrome, a disorder of the heart's electrical system. Parkinson's other contributions included work on myocardial infarction, angina pectoris, and the importance of radiology in cardiac diagnosis. He was a mentor to many younger cardiologists, and used his leadership position to promote international cardiology, along with White.

Bedford (1898–1978) was a pioneer in the study of myocardial infarction with Parkinson. He was also an expert on atrial septal defects and their repair, and helped discover the cause of pulmonary congestion. An encyclopedic mind, he was devoted to the history of cardiology. He was a highly literate and well-traveled man who sometimes worked with a cigarette stub dangling from his lip.

As for Wood (1907–1962), he was born in the hill-station of Coonoor, India, where his father was posted as a British civil servant. He was one of the first to measure intravascular pressures and oxygen saturation in patients with congenital and valvular heart disease, providing a scientific basis for surgical correction. He introduced rigorous bed-side diagnostic methods, and was committed to confirmation of clinical findings by cardiac catheterization. He was also well-known for his textbook derived from personal experience, *Diseases of the Heart and Circulation* (which he dedicated to Parkinson). Wood was fond of dazzling postgraduate students like us, as well as visitors, with his riveting bedside diagnoses.

Studying for the MRCP also meant working at several hospitals to which we were posted by turns. The first was the National Hospital, Queensway, where I came across excellent neurology clinicians such as Sir Francis Walshe (1885–1973), Macdonald Critchley (1900–1997), and Swithin Meadows (1902–1993), who were very inspiring and helped enhance my knowledge of neurology. My next posting was to the Brompton Hospital for chest diseases, this was also highly clinical. The third posting was to the Hospital for Skin Diseases which was dominated by the clinical acumen of Dr. R.M.B. MacKenna (1903–1984). In short, chest diseases, heart disease, neurology and skin dominated our studies. In those days, there was very little technology and good clinical acumen was stressed by all our teachers.

The other foreign postgraduate students in the UK came from the other British colonies. While Australia, New Zealand, Canada, and South

Africa contributed a few, the majority were from India, Pakistan, and Sri Lanka, with the remainder coming from Syria, Egypt, Iraq, Hong Kong, and Singapore. There were none from the USA. Today, most medical students take their postgraduate examinations in their own countries, and do not care to take the MRCP. The only persons taking the MRCP these days are foreign nationals who are residents of the U.K. We all took the exam together and that made for great companionship.

London had only recently come through the war years. Living there was often uncomfortable and cold. There was no central heating, and we had to rely on shilling-operated gas heaters. I stayed with two landladies one after the other and ate bad vegetarian British food, but I had great freedom of movement. I made a lot of Indian and other Colonial friends by taking the same courses, and also befriended other Indians who were fellow boarders, people such as Dr. Coluthur Gopalan (later Director-General of the Indian Council of Medical Research).

The weather in England is proverbial except in some cases in the summer, and clouds, rains and fog are the usual forecast. In spite of this, I visited all the tourist spots, including Hampton Court, the Tower of London, and of course Westminster Abbey and Buckingham Palace. I was in London in 1947 when the Queen got married, and although I have not met her personally, I saw her at close quarters during her wedding, and she looked spectacular then, at the age of 21! I also went to watch Wimbledon and enjoyed it. Outside London, I made a point of visiting places associated with my favourite authors, including the Lake District (Wordsworth, Ruskin, and Beatrix Potter), Stratford on Avon (Shakespeare), Ayot St Lawrence (George Bernard Shaw), and Abbotsford (Sir Walter Scott). I also traveled to the continent, touring France and Switzerland.

At Edinburgh, where I obtained another MRCP which was elevated in due course to FRCP, I came across two other clinical giants: Andrew Gilchrist and Sir Ian Hill. They were general physicians with cardiology as a special area of interest. Gilchrist (1899–1995) was the earliest to diagnose myocardial infarctions, and also recorded the first seven cases of coronary thrombosis in Europe. He carried out fundamental work on anticoagulants, cardiac arrhythmias, paediatric cardiology and cardiac problems in pregnancy. He was a huge Scotsman with an intimidating appearance but with an excellent sense of humour. Hill (1904–1982) was known for his work on electrocardiography with Frank Wilson in Ann Arbor, Michigan and C.J. Rothberger in Vienna, and was responsible for bringing the latest electrocardiographic technology to Britain. He had served in India and Burma during the war and had several Indian postgraduate students.

Sweden

I went to Sweden after my MRCP for a short stint as it was then reputed to be an advanced centre for cardiology. I went to the Karolinska Institute to work with Dr. Gunnar Björck (1916–1996), who later became well-known as Sweden's foremost cardiologist. Subsequently I also worked with Dr. Gustav Nylin (1892–1961) in his private clinic. Nylin was well-known for his groundbreaking studies of blood circulation. Through my interactions with all the professors, I learnt a lot about new technology. The language was no problem, as most Swedes spoke English.

Björck and Nylin were very good to me and from them I learnt a lot about medicine as well as the country's culture. Both were very kind to invite me to their homes. I enjoyed the smorgasbord (a type of meal of hot and cold dishes, typical of the region). I had the pleasure of learning much of Nordic history relating to the Vikings, Uppsala (home of the oldest university in Scandinavia, and once an ancient centre for worship of the Norse Gods), and the Kalmar Union (when Norway, Denmark, Sweden, and Iceland were ruled by a single monarch). During my stay in the country, I also found time to visit Norway and Denmark, and some of the hospitals in these countries. I also saw the Northern Lights and plenty of reindeer.

United States of America

My first fellowship in the US was in 1949 in paediatric cardiology at the Johns Hopkins Hospital in Baltimore. Helen Taussig (1898–1986) was the chief of paediatric cardiology there, while Alfred Blalock (1899–1964) was the chief cardiac surgeon. Denton Cooley (1920–2016) was also there, as a surgical resident. It was here that I witnessed a heart surgery performed by the renowned Blalock, whose work with Taussig on the 'Blue Baby syndrome' went on to shape the future of cardiac surgery and mark a beginning of an era in modern medicine. The Blue Baby operation had been done there for the first time only a few years before I joined, and the hospital's Harriet Lane Home was full of children with the syndrome, seeking surgery from all over the world. Subsequently I saw procedures performed by eminent surgeons such as Donald Ross (1922–2014), who was later to perform the UK's first heart transplant, Michael DeBakey (1908–2008) and Sir Magdi Yacoub. DeBakey was the inventor of the roller pump, an essential component of the heart-lung machine, and one of the first to perform bypass surgery and he also carried out the first patch-graft angioplasty, with his grafts now in standard use all over the world. As for Yacoub, he was an Egyptian Christian who moved to the UK where he became a leader in heart transplantation. He is currently Professor of Cardiothoracic Surgery at Imperial College, London. I also worked at Johns Hopkins with Richard Bing (1909–2010), a pioneer in research into cardiac metabolism. Bing was something of a polymath, publishing more than 500 academic works along with 300 works of music and five works of fiction!

The care and the diligence involved in all these surgeries, coupled with the concern projected by the surgeons and anaesthesiologists involved impressed me greatly. Apart from this, the use of the then-latest equipment, such as heart–lung machines (which required a separate team of analysts) also left a deep impression on me.

I stayed at the nurses' hostel at John Hopkins throughout my stay. It was not very comfortable but close enough for me to go early to work. I played tennis at Hopkins and also spent weekends with my friends in Baltimore. It was a very pleasant stay and I worked very hard. Helen Taussig used to invite us to her home for dinner and lunch parties and once to her summer home in Cotuit, Massachusetts where we could swim the Atlantic and also run around New England. An old friend of hers, Betty Bopp, did all the cooking. A girl from Holland by the name of Van Walbeek was also my companion during this trip, and together, we explored New England and had a very good time. Dr. Taussig was a very good hostess, and gave us good American food. Dr. Taussig remained a lifelong friend and visited me as a house guest in Delhi several times, while also teaching our students at Lady Hardinge Medical College. She was one of the chief guests at the Fifth World Congress of Cardiology and her lecture there on congenital defects was outstanding. I will return to her in Chapter Five (Offshoots of Professional Life).

In 1952, I went on to a fellowship at Harvard University at the Massachusetts General Hospital under Paul Dudley White (1886–1973), which was equally exciting. White was an institution himself at Harvard and is widely regarded as the founder of preventive cardiology. Dr. White and Dr. Taussig have been my gurus ever since. During my stay, I also had the chance to meet and hear stalwarts such as Andre Cournand (1895–1988), who later went on to share the Nobel Prize for his work on cardiac catheterization, and many other celebrities of the time at the Brigham Children Hospital, New England Deaconess Hospital (Boston) and the Mayo Clinic.

As a result of the time I spent in the country, the US became my second home, which I have frequently visited since Dr. Paul White also became a lifelong friend as did his wife, whom I used to visit after Dr. White passed away. Dr. White had many Indian patients, and an account of his visit to India is also given in Chapter Five.

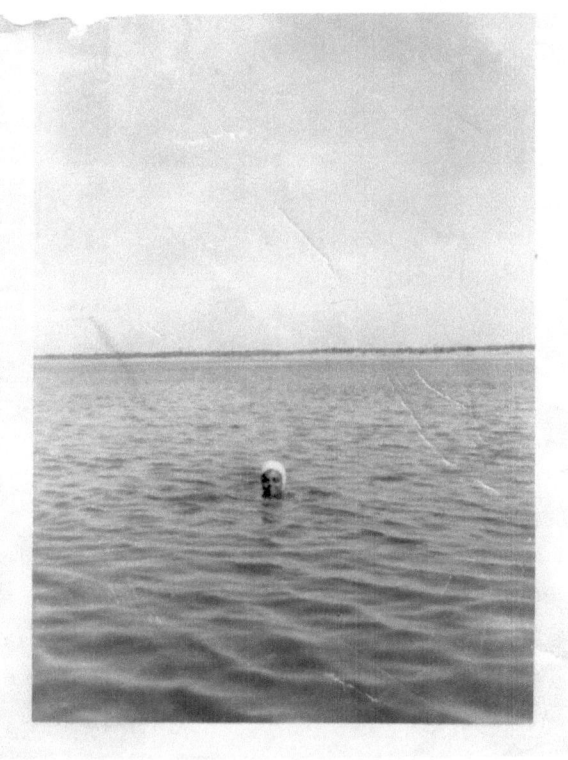

Swimming in the Atlantic at Cotuit

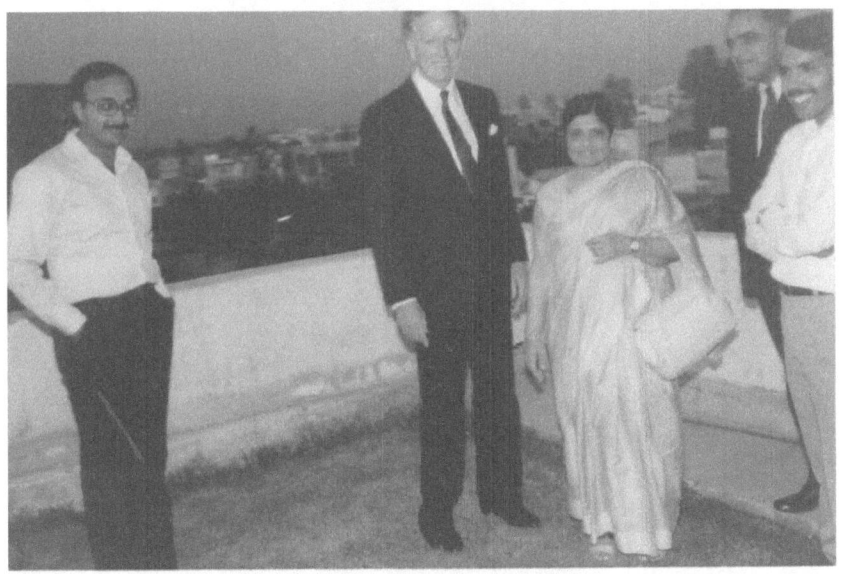

With Dr. Denton Cooley

Chapter 4
Professional Life

Lady Hardinge Medical College

After my post graduate-studies in the West were completed, I went to Burma but could not find any posts suited to my qualifications. I then returned to India. My decision to return was largely influenced by my desire to spend time with my parents in the sunset years of their lives. I was naturally attached to them and wanted to be with them as they aged. Within two years of my return, in 1954, my father died. I was grief-stricken but spared the guilt of not having spent time with him in his last days. I wouldn't have done things differently and am glad that I came back on my own accord.

When I returned to India, with no roots in the country, my first port of call was Delhi, where Rajkumari Amrit Kaur—the first Health minister of free India—offered me the job of a lecturer in medicine at the Lady Hardinge Medical College (LHMC). I took the job after some hesitation, as I suspected I was being relegated to a women's institution on account of my gender. However, I was pleasantly surprised by the atmosphere there. The LHMC had been run by the Women's Medical Service before independence as an all-women college, with absolutely no men students. Except for two male professors in Physiology and Pathology, all the teachers were also women. I found the Department of Medicine orderly, with an early version of an ECG machine. It required the patient to have both feet and a hand in buckets of salt water.

The standard leads (the only ones available those days) were recorded on glass plates and neatly stored away.

Paediatrics in those days was not a separate division. The wards were full of young female patients with Rheumatic Heart Disease (RHD), and children with Acute Rheumatic Fever (RF), some as young as three. I had left the US just as RF/RHD clinics were shutting down and was very surprised at the scenario in India. Thus began my interest in RF/RHD. Cor pulmonale was another area of concern to me at LHMC, with the hospital seeing many cases of young women admitted with acute congestive cardiac failure. I believe the LHMC was the first medical college to publish an account of this in the journal *Circulation* in 1959 and received universal acclaim. Needless to say, all the articles on Cor pulmonale produced by the college were written jointly with my female colleagues in the Department of Medicine and published in journals of repute. My colleagues at the department of Medicine at Lady Harding were Drs. S.N. Pathak (deceased), Savitri Gupta, Santosh Sood, Saroj Kumari, Kasturi Agarwal (deceased), Veena Raizada, Ramesh Arora, Indrajit Sandhu and the ECG technician who was a multi-purpose member of the team, A. Kalawati (deceased) .

As the only medical college in the federal capital, LHMC was pampered a great deal. Many important visitors to Delhi made a point of making a stop at the college, and gave lectures and suggestions. Notable among them were Princess Lilliane of Belgium, the Yugoslavian heart surgeon Dr. Izidor Papo, who was surgeon to President Josip Broz Tito of Yugoslavia, Dr. Doyle of Australia and Dr. Michael DeBakey from the US. Soon, research grants began to pour in, from the World Health Organization (WHO), US Public Health Service, programs to implement Public Law 480 (the U.S. Agricultural Trade Development and Assistance Act of 1954), Department of Science and Technology, India, and the Indian Council of Medical Research. It was a great source of inspiration for the staff and students.

The first cheque for RF/RHD was handed to me by Mrs. Chester Bowles, wife of the American Ambassador. The first cardiac clinic in North India was started at the LHMC in 1954, and the first cardiac catheterization lab in North India was setup in the college in 1954, with equipment donated by the Rockefeller Foundation. Today, the cardiac catheterization process has been simplified by the arrival of catheters that record oxygen saturation and more sophisticated X-Ray machines. But the equipment sent to LHMC was of the older type, and in keeping with the kind I had worked with at Johns Hopkins under Dr. Richard Bing. The Rockefeller Foundation, however, sent us machines that suited our purpose of studying Cor pulmonale effectively and coming up with groundbreaking research in the field. The clinic became very popular, seeing a large number of cases of congenital heart disease and RHD, and also some cases of coronary heart disease. Soon male physicians were seeking out work in our cardiac catheterization lab, demonstrating that even in those early days in India, women's colleges and hospitals could lead the way. Meanwhile, many of the old-timers resented the presence of men in the campus, but their voices were not heard.

The first Patent Ductus Arteriosus (PDA) ligation was performed by Dr. Papo in 1957 on an LHMC patient, during the peak of the Non-aligned Movement. Considering the prominence of LHMC, it is then not surprising to note that the All India Heart Foundation was inaugurated at the LHMC in 1962, with participation from eminent people in the field from all across India.

The LHMC campus, incidentally, had two tennis courts and one swimming pool, which I thoroughly enjoyed. Recently, at the centennial celebrations in 2016, when I went there as a Guest of Honour, the only thing I could recognize was the statue of Lady Hardinge, as everything else had been changed. There were many more buildings, students' and nurses' hostels and homes for the doctors. No doubt, it was necessary, but it spoilt the look of the place.

Princess Lilliane's husband, King Leopold III of Belgium, presented me with his book on the tribes of Andaman, which I treasure to this day. Lilliane invited me to the palace in Brussels, and I eventually managed a visit. I learnt a lot of European history in my time there, including the story of the loss of Europe to the Turks.

GB Pant Hospital and Maulana Azad Medical College

In 1967, I moved to the newly formed G. B. Pant Hospital for super specialties as Director and Consultant in cardiology. Soon after I joined, I was given an additional role, taking over from Dr. Pathak who had gone on leave, as Director-Principal of Maulana Azad Medical College (MAMC). The latter was one unit, with the Pant and Lok Nayak Jai Prakash Narayan Hospitals (LNH, earlier Irwin Hospital) under its care. The Guru Nanak Eye Centre had just been added to this list. It was a very interesting time with so many heads of departments working together (25 in all). One had the chance to learn a lot from their experiences as most of them were extremely dedicated to their subjects. It had Cardiology, Cardiac Surgery, Neurology, Neuro-Surgery, Gastroenterology, and Psychiatry. I was the head of both Pant Hospital and also the departments of Cardiology and Cardiac Surgery.

The Directorship of MAMC included not only the college, but also the Directorship of LNH. When I left MAMC in 1977, the post of Director-Principal was replaced by that of Dean. Since then, all the institutions are autonomous, including the new Dental sciences one. I do not know whether this is a better arrangement, because in my time, it was easy to post students across institutions, and frequent meetings helped create a sense of camaraderie. The annual sports function and the annual convocation were occasions when the entire staff from all the institutions would come together and get a chance to mingle. It was a very busy and exciting time. We interacted freely and regularly with other developing centres at Vellore and Bombay.

When I joined Pant Hospital, it was a real challenge to set up the new department. However, the support of an enthusiastic staff made it possible, and we were soon up and running. My colleagues there were Dr. N.S. Dixit (deceased), Dr. G.D. Gupta, Dr. M.P. Gupta (deceased), and Dr. M. Khalilullah, who remained fast friends of mine. It was in this role that my knowledge of cardiology truly expanded as the field was witnessing significant development of new drugs, new technology, neurophysiology and cardiac surgery. I was always travelling to Cardiology conferences as it was an opportune time for Cardiology to develop.

Pant Hospital is an establishment that can boast of many firsts in medicine in North India. The first pacemaker implant surgery was carried out in 1960, the first coronary care unit (CCU) of the region was inaugurated in 1971, and the first EPS (Electrophysiology) study was undertaken in 1972. The Doctor of Medicine, Doctor of Cardiology and Master of Chirurgical, Cardiothoracic and Vascular Surgery degrees were offered for the first time in 1960. Several union government ministers, such as the Finance and Planning Minister C. Subramaniam, the ministers and diplomats D.P. Dhar and the (very contentious) V.K. Krishna Menon were treated for heart ailments at the hospital. Prime Minister Indira Gandhi was also a frequent visitor. After Shri Dhar developed V-tach in 1972 at the Simla Summit (which was also visited by Pakistan President Zulfikar Ali Bhutto), he was airlifted to Pant Hospital.

The following is an article I had written on my experience of the Simla Summit, reproduced in full.

Kargil and the Simla Summit

Kargil is hot news these days. The media and the public are harking back to the Simla Accord of 1972, when firm foundations were laid for Indo–Pak amity. Kargil is now considered a travesty of this accord. My own small involvement in this historic event is the subject of this article.

It was around 4 a.m on the morning of 1st July 1972, when my bedside telephone rang shrilly and non-stop. A voice at the other end said, "Madam, you are wanted immediately in Simla. Mr. D.P. Dhar is very ill. A car will pick you up for the morning flight to Chandigarh shortly!" I had barely put the receiver down when the car arrived. I hastily got dressed and caught the early morning flight. On arrival in Chandigarh, an army helicopter was waiting for me. We landed at the improvised helipad at Simla, only to be whisked away in a waiting car to Snowdon Hospital, where Mr. Dhar had been shifted the previous night.

Mr. Dhar was the key negotiator at the Simla summit. He had had an acute myocardial infarction in Moscow a while ago and had been receiving treatment at GB Pant Hospital. At the moment, he was stable, but he had had an alarming attack of sudden tachycardia the evening before after some hectic parleying. Dr. K.P. Mathur—the Prime Minister's physician—and local doctors had been called to attend on him and the attack had subsided. After that, he had been shifted to the Snowdon Hospital. The attack was diagnosed as ventricular tachycardia. As the hospital had very few facilities, a monitor and technician had to be brought in from PGI Chandigarh to continuously monitor his condition.

Come to think of it, the facilities those days by way of equipment or drugs, especially at Simla, were appalling, particularly when compared with today's plethora of both. There was no Amiodarone, no Xylocard, no pacing catheters, no echocardiograph, no Holter and no telemetry; only old-style defibrillators were available. With a little luck and a few old-fashioned drugs, the patient made an uneventful recovery. He was ambulated to the monitor through a long cord around the ward. He was, however, extremely cheerful and co-operative and this contributed to the quick improvement.

I saw a lot of Mrs. Gandhi then, as she was in and out of the hospital. What struck me about her was the extremely matter-of-fact attitude towards the whole episode and complete confidence in the doctors. I also caught glimpses of Mr. Zulfikar Ali Bhutto, who I thought was rather flamboyantly dressed. Benazir was also there, a young girl and not yet as glamorous as she would later be. I remember that Mr. Dhar presented her with a beautiful Shatoosh shawl.

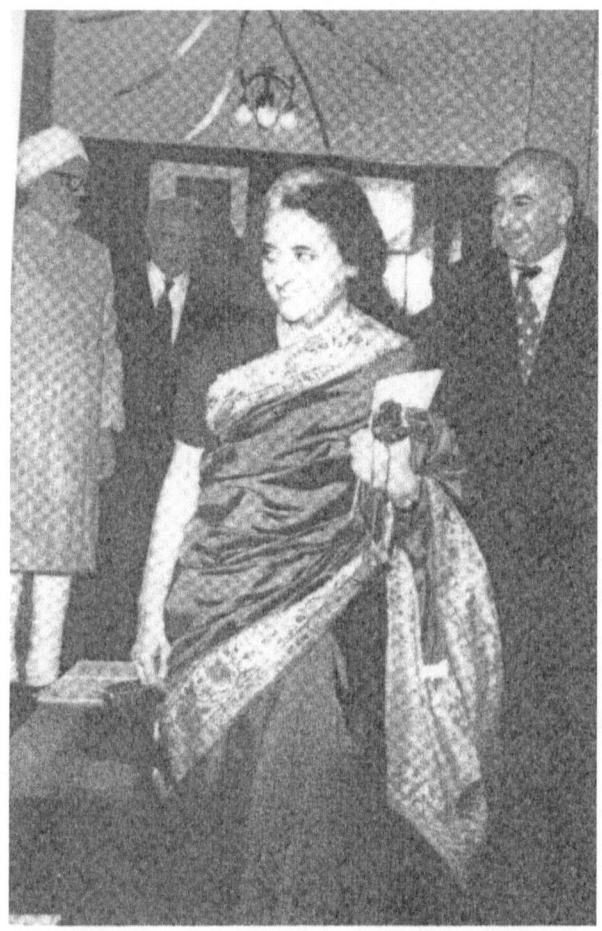

Indira Gandhi with Zulfikar Bhutto, Simla Summit

I stayed at the Cecil along with the other delegates. Because I had left in such a hurry and not had time to pack, I had to wear clothes belonging to the hotel manager's wife, who was about the same build and size as me.

After a few days, it was decided that Mr. Dhar would be taken back to Delhi, as he was fit to travel. We reached the helipad with top army brass, including General Candeth, in attendance. The army paramedics on the helicopter were extremely efficient, and we reached Chandigarh after a smooth flight. Contrastingly, the ride in the special government plane that took us to Delhi was rather bumpy. Mr. Dhar stood both flights very well. It was nice to get back to the reassuring safety and efficiency of the G.B. Pant

Hospital, which was a well-equipped cardiac centre by the standards of that time. We received many congratulatory telegrams and letters from all over India at Mr. Dhar's safe transfer from Chandigarh. The Simla summit had naturally made headline news. It really was an extremely memorable visit.

Mr. Dhar was nursed back to good health at the G.B. Pant Hospital and lived to hold important cabinet posts until his terminal illness in 1975. But that is another story.

A rather odd incident occurred in 1971, while I was at MAMC and Pant. A gentleman by the name of Rustom Sohrab Nagarwala, a former Army intelligence officer, had apparently called up the State Bank of India and impersonated Prime Minister Indira Gandhi's voice, demanding a withdrawal of sixty lakh rupees, to be handed over to a Bangladeshi. (India was at the time supporting freedom fighters in Bangladesh.) Upon dispensing the amount, the bank official was told to go to the PM's office to collect the receipt, whereupon the fraud was discovered. Nagarwala was arrested, and shortly after, was admitted to Irwin hospital with a heart complaint. I used to see him there on my rounds, until he suddenly died. Given that the investigating officer also died, in a car crash, the Opposition cried foul, saying Mrs. Gandhi's hand was behind the fraud and accused her of arranging for a technician from GB Pant hospital to kill Nagarwala. However, a routine biopsy by the head of Autopsy found evidence of severe heart disease, with the doctor preserving the heart to show to students. The machinations involved in the fraud remain a mystery, but regarding the cause of death, the conclusion was clear.

All India Heart Foundation and National Heart Institute

I became involved with the All India Heart Foundation (AIHF) in 1962 and played an active role in its development after I retired. The AIHF was founded in 1962 with Dr. Paul White as the main inspiration and many doctors and business executives from all over India participated in its opening. Prominent among them were Shri Lakshmipat Singhania, Dr. J.C. Bannerjee, Dr. K.K. Datey and Dr. Ratnavelu Subramanyam. It became a very active collaborative centre of the WHO for 29 years and contributed actively to public health education, research, training of doctors and paramedics, and population outreach.

The AIHF celebrated its Golden Jubilee in August 2010. Over the years, it has organized conferences such as the First World Congress of Cardiology in 1966, the Indo-American conference on Rheumatic Fever in 1981, and the first Asian-Pacific conference of Cardiology in 2004. It has distributed free pacemakers and ICDs to about 125 poor patients a year, obtained from Heartbeat International of the USA. (I joined Heartbeat thanks to my friendship with the late Dr. Henry McIntosh, who helped found it, as I thought it was a wonderful opportunity to help poor patients.) The AIHF also arranges heart camps to increase awareness of heart disease, which is after all the number one killer in India. The foundation celebrates World Heart Day, World No Tobacco Day, and Diabetes Day with free heart camps, exhibitions and dialogues with the public. World Heart Day, in particular, is a big affair, with a Walkathon, dialogue with the public both in the morning and evening, along with a Question and Answer session in the afternoon at the India International Centre (of which it is now a corporate member). These events have been well attended and souvenirs are published after each event.

Because of land sold at low rates by the Delhi Government, the National Heart Institute (NHI) was built at a cost of Rs 1.5 crore in 1981 and inaugurated by Mrs. Indira Gandhi. It was the first Heart Institute in India as well as in Asia. Today, there are nearly 100 institutes and cardiac centres in the country. The institution has grown over the years and now holds a hundred beds, as opposed to the twenty it housed when founded. It also trains doctors and paramedics in cardiology and ancillary disciplines. The second phase of development of NHI was inaugurated by K.R. Narayanan, Vice-President of India and later President. The NHI celebrated its Silver Jubilee in 2006, a remarkable success story given the competition from private hospitals. Unlike the latter, the NHI depends on aid, which can help it develop even further.

I have to mention three administrators who were responsible for the growth of the AIHF and NHI. These were Mr. R. Ramamirtham, first Secretary of the AIHF, Mr. N. Venkatraman, Secretary and Mr. P. C. Jain, administrator of the NHI, who have now all passed away. My colleagues at the AIHF and NHI have been Dr. Vinod Sharma, Dr. L.C. Gupta, Dr. A.P. Arora on the medical side, and Dr. O.P. Yadava on the surgical side.

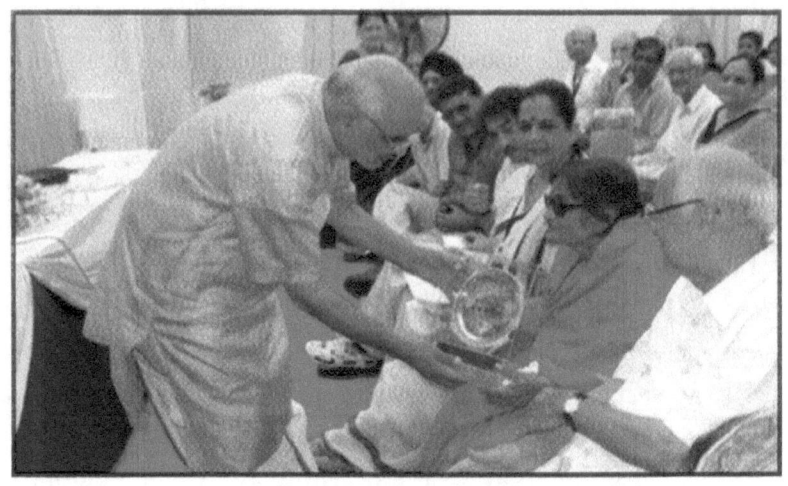

Silver Jubilee Receiving Award Dr. S. Janaki

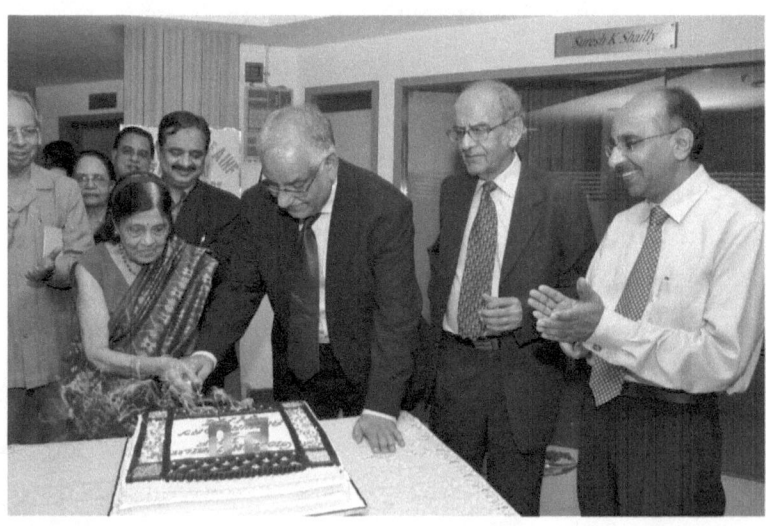

Golden Jubilee Dr. S. Padmavati & Prof G N Quazi V C Jamia Hamdard

Fifth World Congress of Cardiology

The Fifth World Congress of Cardiology helped place India on the world cardiology map. It was held in 1966, for the first and only time in India, under the auspices of the AIHF and World Heart Federation. It was hosted at Vigyan Bhawan, the state of the art government building for conferences at that time and was thus supported in many ways by the government. The following is an excerpt of my recollection of the event.

The Fifth World Congress of Cardiology was one of the major seminars, held by the AIHF and CSI in Delhi. All doctors and their wives flocked to Delhi in the November of 1966 in warm weather that wasn't at all oppressive. The impressive auditorium of Vigyan Bhawan was the site of the inauguration of the event. At the opening event, the participants were honoured by the presence of the country's then President Dr. S. Radhakrishnan, who in his address underlined the importance of cardiology not only as a vast clinical specialty but also in relation to world health.

In his gracious speech, Dr. K.K. Datey, the president of the congress, outlined the work that was to be done in the country. He also referred to learning that could be derived from India's heritage and seeing other parts of the land. The congress was acclaimed by all sides as an unqualified success. This was the result of a long and exacting planning of the event by Dr. Datey and the secretary general, Padmavati. Besides the flow of events, we had also kept in mind the comfort and enjoyment of the participants, hospitality to the members and the success of these events in the day-to-day organisation of the congregation. These efforts were widely appreciated. We had also planned entertainment for the wives and family members, hence making it a satisfying experience for them.

At meetings of the Council and the General Assembly, some important decisions were made. Sir Kempson Maddox was elected President of the International Society to succeed Dr. Pierre Duchosal, who had conducted the affairs of the society with outstanding success before this. Far-sighted developments were planned for the field of science. The event was grouped into eight sections—atherosclerosis and ischaemic heart disease, clinical electro-physiology, epidemiology and preventive cardiology, hypertension, rehabilitation, cardiomyopathies and paediatric cardiology. Each section was responsible for coordinating, on a global basis, research, training and education in its own particular discipline. From Britain, M.F. Oliver of Edinburgh and Hamish Watson of Dundee, were appointed heads of the section of atherosclerosis and paediatric cardiology, respectively.

A symposium, which had been planned with much care and forethought, was held each morning. In general, these were highly successful and provoked useful discussion. No simultaneous meetings were held during these occasions, and the result was an auditorium filled almost to capacity, with none of the exchange or attenuation among the audience that can be so distracting to speaker and hearer alike. Some of the meetings in subsidiary halls in the afternoon attracted much larger audiences than were expected, and on a few of these occasions, even standing room was limited. The system of multiple small afternoon meetings had the advantage of more informal discussion, but inevitably meant that some good papers were presented simultaneously. The need to accept enough contributions to satisfy national aspirations and at the same time avoid overcrowding of sessions and too many simultaneous sessions is an ever recurring difficulty for congress organisers and present increasing problems for those who plan such congresses.

Notable among the many worth-while contributions were the sessions allotted to the assessment by physicians of the effects of cardiac surgery, the paper on treatment of tricuspid defects at mitral valve replacement and in Ebstein's disease, and a good double-blind study showing the effect of the use of anticoagulants in myocardial infarction. Papers on heart surgery showed improved operative results in transposition and discussed the place of total correction in the tetralogy of Fallot and the value of corrective operations on the mitral and aortic valves. There were no sessions on coronary heart disease surgery or stents or on angioplasty.

The congress was notable for the lavish entertainment offered to visitors. Performances of ethnic music and dancing, and of ballet in the open air were unforgettable, and on a more personal level, the many garden parties and evening functions provided relaxation from the arduous professional work. The congress evening party held under a vast and resplendent shamiana *was also outstanding. Concourses on this scale are in a different category from the meetings of small groups of experts to discuss a defined problem. The latter deal more with the growing points in cardiology science, while the former foster international friendships as well as provide a survey of cardiology work in a great variety of disciplines, and are valuable for those whose work takes them more to the bedside than to the laboratory. For some, the conclusion of the congress was the starting point of visits to Ceylon or Rajasthan. Others converged at New Delhi after travelling to Nepal or Kashmir. For all, there were indelible memories of the warm welcome of their hosts, the reunion of old friends and the innumerable and vivid impressions made by this land, with its heritage of ancient art culture.*

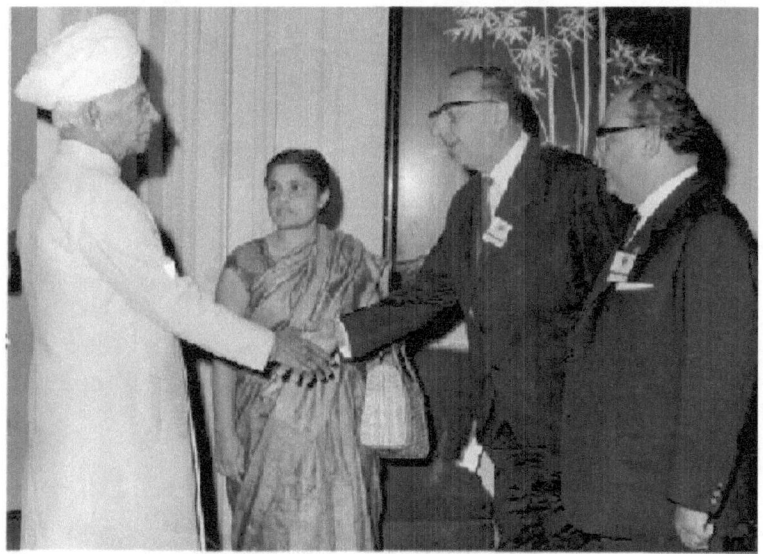

Dr. S. Radhakrishanan Meeting Guests and Participants.

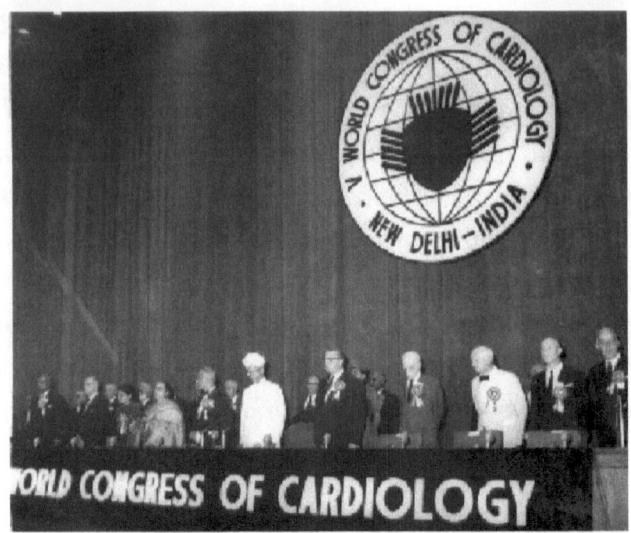

Seminar at the Opening Ceremony

India in those days was considered a very remote country full of fakirs and elephants and very difficult to approach. When the conference was so well conducted and organized, the delegates were pleasantly surprised! Among the events at the Congress was the birth of the International Society for Cardiology's Scientific Council on Epidemiology and Prevention, described in this colorful eyewitness account from the University of Minnesota:

A huge, brightly colored tent, festooned with flowing banners and lit by flaming tapers, covered a large area adjacent to the Hotel Ashoka and housed the opening reception and banquet of the World Congress of Cardiology in New Delhi in fall 1966. Steaming tables of saffron rice and roast chicken, endless varieties of legumes and vegetables, and groaning boards of sweets tempted the delegates gathered in the exotic setting. The main organizational business of the congress would include formation of the International Society's eight new scientific councils, including the Council on Epidemiology and Prevention. After twelve years of planning and politicking by White, Keys, and colleagues, the new council was formally charged with the development of standard field methods and criteria, of training programs for researchers, of collaborative population studies and prevention trials, and of public-policy recommendations for CVD prevention.

Thus, the festive opening of the congress was full of promise for the preventionists. Unhappily, in the days immediately following the grand reception, many delegates found themselves ill-adapted to the exotic cuisine and their organizational tasks had to be borne by those few who remained upright and vigorous. The minutes of the organizational meeting in New Delhi included two ideas forming the framework of the new Council's intent. The first was "recognition that a key strategy in the control of epidemic cardiovascular disease–particularly coronary heart disease–was primary prevention." A second was based on the observation that incidence of these diseases varied greatly among the world's populations, and that "study of the factors related to these differences–that is, epidemiological investigations–could help form the necessary scientific foundation for prevention".

Observations on Health Care for the Masses

India is a land of 1.3 billion people, with a substantial portion mired in poverty. Providing health care to such a large population spread across different social classes is an enormous challenge. Having worked in both the public and the private sectors, I have noticed that the private sector, which now provides over 85% of tertiary health care, is very different from the government-run hospitals. Private hospitals do not see the variety of diseases one sees in free government hospitals and they mostly treat patients with coronary artery disease and hypertension. In government-run hospitals, in contrast, I have observed a wider range of heart diseases across all social groups. It is for this reason that I advise young doctors and aspiring cardiologists to serve in the public sector for a part of their careers. This can help equip them better to deal with a variety of heart diseases.

Of course, the private sector also has much better equipment, better maintenance and better standards of hygiene. If the poor are to be treated in these hospitals, then costs need to be regulated like they are in Singapore, instead of the government trying to improve old government hospitals. What is required in the current economy is that the private and public sectors engage in earnest and arrive at an agreement, instead of indulging in acrimonious debate.

Cardiology in India has really come of age much more so than in other developing countries of Asia, Africa and Latin America. But what bothers me is the unequal distribution of healthcare. With 40% to 70% of the population (the figures are disputed) below the poverty line and without access to any kind of medical aid, how can all these wonderful developments reach the common man? Other drawbacks of the current system are lack of research, insufficient manpower—both of doctors and paramedics—poor infrastructure and insufficient medical care for children. The government's efforts, laudable on paper, are often mired in corruption during implementation. Hence, it is for doctors and the thinking public to find a way.

Another factor affecting advanced medical care is medical tourism. Many cardiac centres and private hospitals have begun to follow the trend of filling hospital beds with people from other countries. The industry of medical tourism is now an extremely large and also lucrative one for private concerns. Sometimes, packages also have an added attraction thrown in, such as tourism after surgery or treatment. Every established hospital today is keen on attracting foreign patients while the poor in India who cannot pay are neglected.

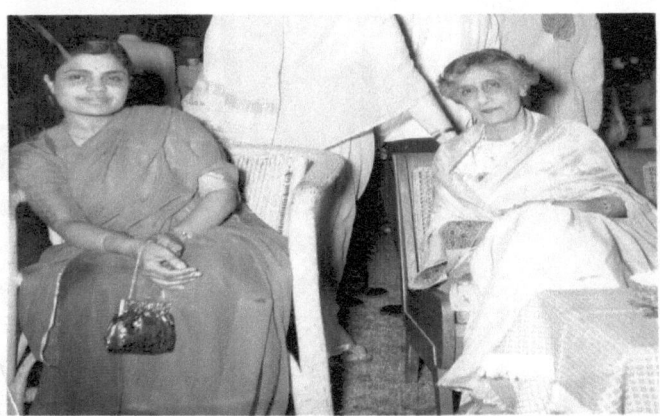

Rajkumari Amrit Kaur

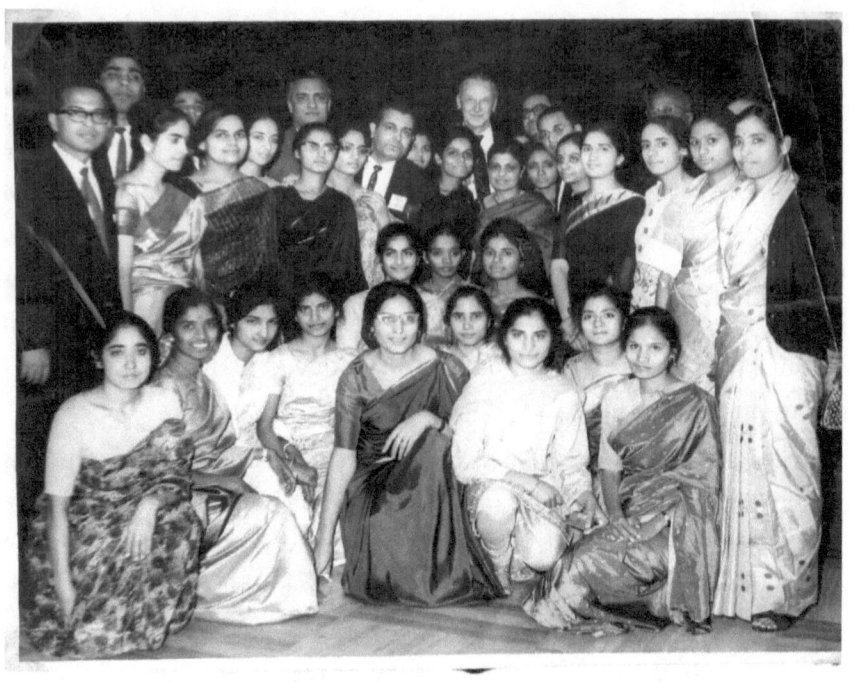

Students at LHMC

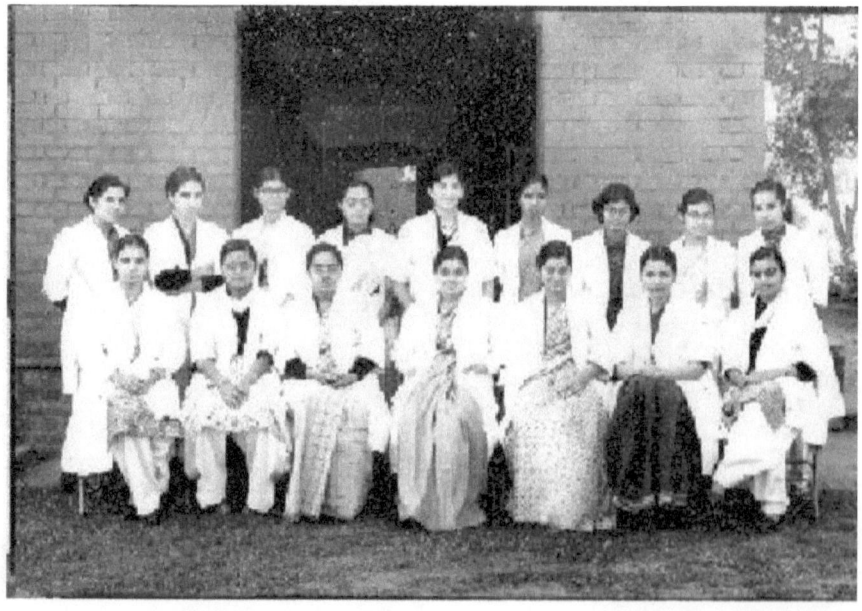

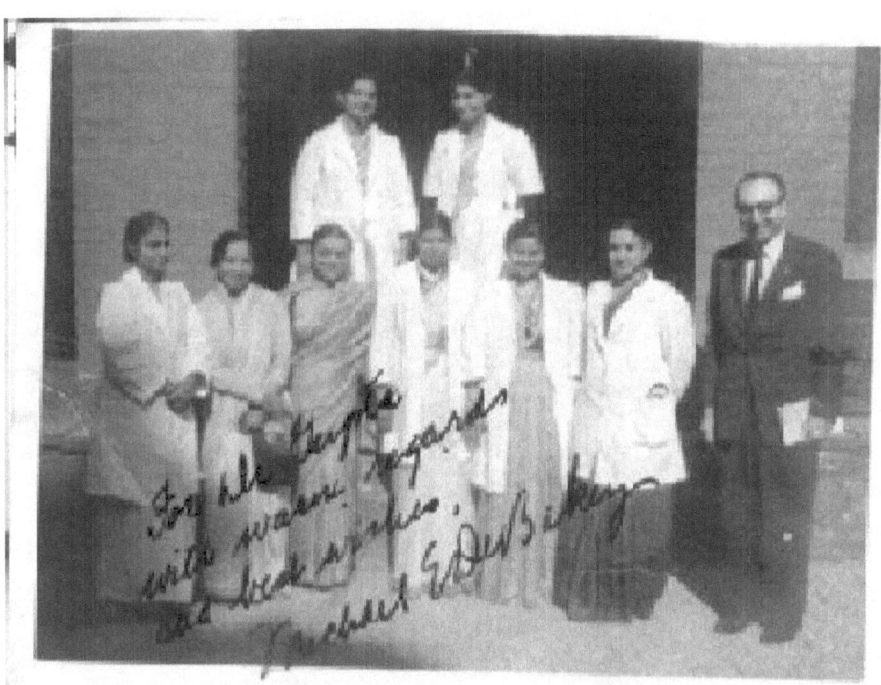

Mike DeBakey at Lady Hardinge

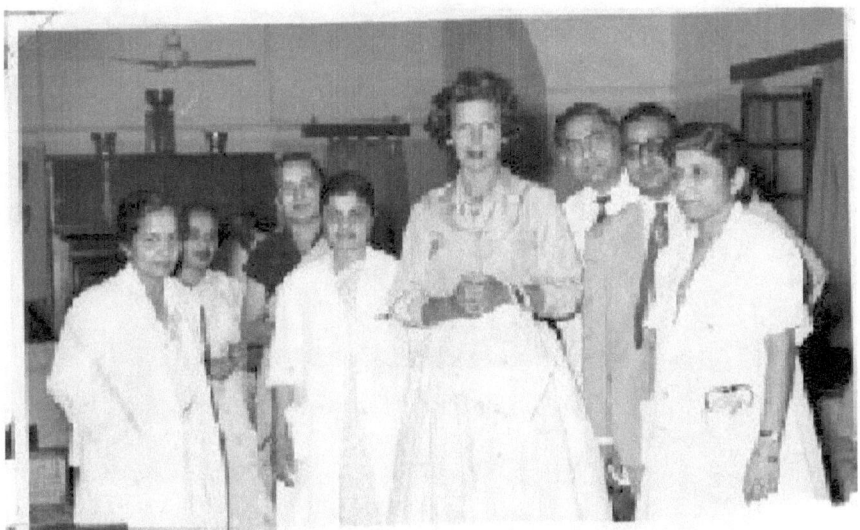

Princess Lilliane with the LHMC Staff

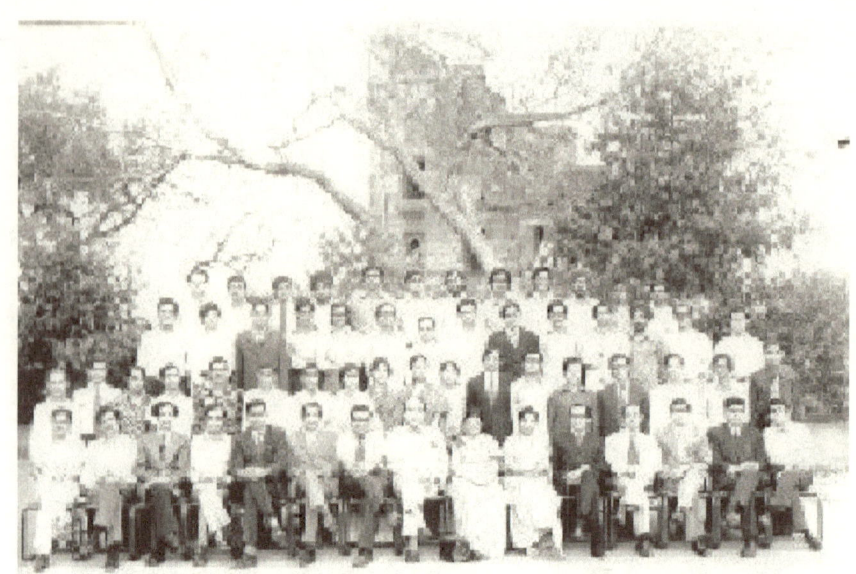

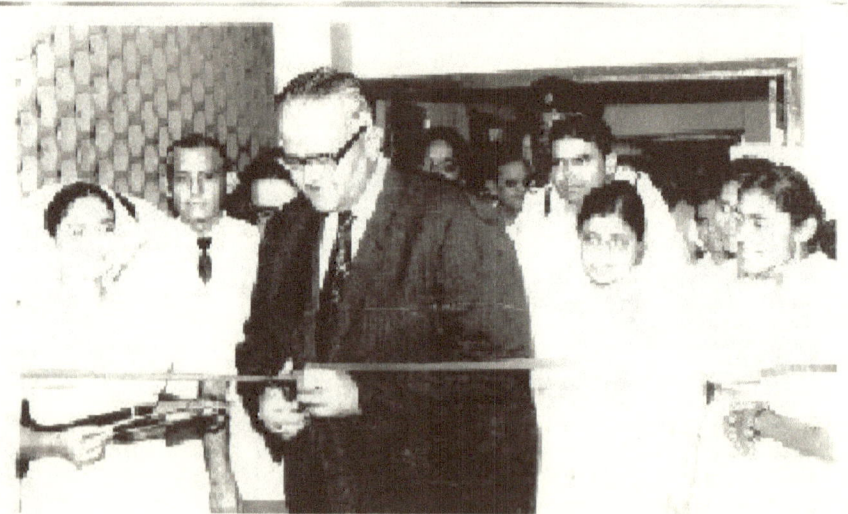

Opening of the CCU at G.B. Pant

Chapter 5
Offshoots of Professional Life

In a career spanning seven decades, I have had many enriching experiences apart from my medical education and practice. Being a medical professional allowed me to pursue expansive research projects and hence contribute to human welfare. Though my work was the most satisfying of all, other offshoots were rewarding too. My travels exposed me to cultures, art and interactions that have significantly moulded my personality and expanded my horizons. The interactions with VIPs and VOPs (Very Ordinary People) added to my medical pursuits and personal experiences. From Blue Bloods to Blue Babies, I have seen all shades of life and cherish my experiences as trophies. People have been kind in recognizing my efforts to nominate me for awards.

Throughout my career, I have been asked repeatedly whether I have faced any discrimination because I am a woman. My answer has always been a resounding NO. Perhaps I was lucky because cardiology had not developed much then, and I was trying to make a breakthrough in the subject. This may be hard to believe, as this is the same country that has a skewed (though diminishing) sex ratio of 933: 1000 in the last census, and is notoriously and regularly in the news because of abortion of female foetuses, ill-treatment of the girl child and of women in general.

Areas of Interest and Contributions

My career has focused on areas such as Preventive Cardiology, International Cardiology, and Cardiovascular Epidemiology.

A core interest of mine has to do with Cor pulmonale in young women. It was one of the first diseases which I had the chance to treat first-hand. I believe we were one of the earliest to report this disease. It started in the LHMC (Lady Hardinge Medical College) and continues till today. At the hospital, the wards were usually full of many young women exhibiting acute symptoms of the disease. Seeing so many people suffer from it had a significant impact and always drove me to work hard to eradicate it. We discovered that the cause of Cor pulmonale in these women was due to their having cooked from an early age over smoky and primitive fireplaces in ill-ventilated huts, damaging their lungs from exposure to smoky cooking fuels. While researching cor pulmonale, I undertook a study of the cause of congestive heart failure among women between the ages of 20 to 30. With the simple tools of ECG, X-rays and clinical examinations available then, in the 1950s, I also identified some of the gases emitted by these stoves. This study went on to prove that the cause for Cor pulmonale among women of this age differed from that among men between 50 to 60 years (which generally resulting from smoking). It was studies like these that led our group at LMHC to become the first to publish on Cor pulmonale in the American journal *Circulation*, in 1959. Our discovery of the cause of cor pulmonale in women was much heralded, even by our male colleagues who had not devoted enough attention to finding the cause! This work points to the importance of lifestyle changes and role of public health in combating heart disease.

Another special area of interest is rheumatic fever (RF) and rheumatic heart disease (RHD). My lifelong interest in RHD began during my fellowship at the Paediatric Cardiac Clinic of Helen Taussig at the John Hopkins Hospital in Baltimore and later grew under Dr. Bernard Masell during a visit to the House of the Good Samaritan in Boston. At Baltimore, I saw many patients suffering from RHD, although the clinic focussed on treating cases of congenital heart disease. In those days, doctors laid the most emphasis on sleeping pulse and ESR, apart from treatment involving penicillin. Patients would be sent to convalescent homes, which Fellows used to visit. Around the late 1950s, most of these homes had shut down because of decline in the disease, attributed to better living conditions and early onset of treatment.

On my return to India, I was struck by the large number of cardiac patients suffering from RHD at Lady Hardinge. What was most alarming was how young the patients were (the youngest was three years old, and presented with florid manifestations) and how severe their conditions were. So much so that the term 'juvenile mitral stenosis' was coined in India. Every cardiac conference of the Cardiology Society of India at that time was concentrated on RHD, its manifestations, prophylaxis and treatment. It was the most common cause of heart disease in most states of India. I believe that my team and I demonstrated conclusively that 3 weekly injections of penicillin were superior to 4 weekly ones in endemic areas. Some more details of our discoveries are described in Chapter 8 (Heart Disease in Neglected Groups).

The Indian Council of Medical Research (ICMR), which was genuinely concerned about the spread of the disease, generously funded research projects on the subject. Following this, there were several collaborative projects with other medical colleges and the WHO. Dr. Tom Strasser was put in charge of all of these. The last projects were the two important integration studies into the Primary Health Centres (PHCs) and the School Health Services (SHS). I was a part of the last one, which concluded in 1990. By that time, in 1984, a streptococcal reference laboratory was also opened in LHMC and also at Christian Medical College, Vellore. It was an integral institution that provided excellent service. Alas, these have now been shut down. Nevertheless, there has been a large amount of research on RHD in this country.

The ICMR undertook two transfers of technology in 1987 and 1994 to propagate the results of these research findings. Although doctors and others involved in RF/RHD and public health workers were all involved, many of the suggested measures were never implemented, as medicine is a prerogative of the States and can only be implemented by the State Government. A 'model' permanent registry at the All India Heart Foundation (AIHF) in Delhi is all that remains of the good intentions of the ICMR. It is disheartening to think that this has featured in only one Five-year Plan (the Fourth) and not since.

On a more positive note, thanks to videos in English, Hindi and Tamil shown at peak viewing hours on Doordarshan, at the initiative of the AIHF and write-ups in English and vernacular newspapers, awareness about RF/RHD increased tremendously in the country. Patients began to seek help wherever it was available. BMV and CMV (closed and open mitral valvotomy, valve replacements and valve repair) were available in the big cities in India, but very few could afford them. Anticoagulation posed its own problems at the time, and the only real solution was prevention. In 1982, at the Ninth World Congress of Preventive Cardiology in Moscow, some of the delegates, including myself, met the Director General of WHO and stressed the importance of RF/RHD control in the greater part of the world. The result was the formation of the Ad Hoc Committee on RF/RHD of the WHF, of which I was a member, which is now a full-fledged council. Some good has resulted from this committee, as some developing countries have set up programs for control of the disease, although with variable results.

I fondly remember my friends Drs. Wannamaker, Rotta, Markowitz and Taranta, who put in a lot of work into mitigating the disease.

We have also shown that RHD can be effectively controlled in primary school children by involving the doctors and nurses of the school health service about the disease. We did a study under the ICMR on 40,000 school children over a period of 5 years. This of course means that the school must have a school health system. At the time of the study, this existed only in Delhi and Madras. Subsequently it has spread to other schools in India although I do not have information about them. As with Cor pulmonale, the research I led on RF/RHD has had substantial public health implications. While I am by no means averse to high-tech innovations, advances in public health need not always depend on these. With the help of school teachers and nurses in the public school to screen and treat children with sore throats, and starting a clinic to give chronic treatment to poor children with heart disease, we were able to save so many lives. While my male colleagues were developing high tech procedures such as bypass and heart transplant that saved relatively few lives, we were able to save millions by empowering women and children.

Cardiovascular epidemiology has been another area of interest. We have published the epidemiology of all kinds of heart disease – congenital, rheumatic, hypertensive and ischaemic. My research in the area of Ischaemic Heart Disease (IHD) helped identify the high risk factors that are commonly detected in India. In this context, I noticed that apart from heredity reasons, hypertension and diabetes seemed to have been more pressing causes than smoking and raised serum cholesterol levels (contrary to the case in Western countries). We have also had the privilege of conducting preventive programmes for IHD with assistance from WHO, which was no mean task at the time. Cardiology being such a new field, especially in India, epidemiology of various heart diseases was still an unexplored field when I began to work on it. I went on to publish my findings in journals of bodies such as WHO, DST and ICMR. I focussed on hypertension, RHD, Cor pulmonale and ischaemic heart disease. I was part of a team that took up a detailed enquiry into the history of hypertension in all Indian states from 1961 onwards, and what we noticed was an increase in hypertension levels from 5 to 30% between then and recent years. We perceived this to be a result of changed habits and lifestyles. From a public health standpoint, we also discerned that educating close relatives and the patients themselves was the best method of controlling this medical condition.

Travels

My work gave me many opportunities to travel and see the world. It was mainly my interest and research in interventional cardiology and epidemiology of RHD that took me to all the continents, except Antarctica.

My travels included trips to Hawaii, Australia, New Zealand and the remote island of Tahiti, where Gauguin (the French artist) did a lot of his work. I particularly enjoyed my visits to South America and Central

America, which included travelling to Machu Pichu, Amazonia, the Patagonian desert and Guatemala.

Mexico has always been one of my favourite destinations, although it is now mired in problems related to smuggling and abuse of narcotic substances. My travels to the country were a memorable experience. What stands out from that trip is my visit to the murals of Diego Riviera. They depicted a timeline of the contributions of people to medicine and development of medical technology that evinced popular ideas and concerns.

I have travelled widely across the US and Canada, and also had the chance to tour Europe. While on the continent, I had the good fortune of visiting the Ashram of Maharishi Mahesh Yogi, which involved crisscrossing across Switzerland by helicopter. I was also fortunate to visit the Russian Federation in its earlier avatar—as the Union of the Soviet Socialist Republics. During my trip, I paid a visit to the museum in Leningrad and many other places, including Tashkent. Over the years, work opportunities made sure that I did not leave Asia unexplored. I visited China, where I met barefoot doctors and gathered hands-on knowledge of traditional systems of medicines through the local people. Japan remains my favourite country, where I travelled from Hokkaido to Kagoshima and saw all the beautiful places. I also visited Indonesia and Thailand at different points in my career.

In 2000, I made my last trip to Burma as a WHO consultant. I was shocked to see the inadequacy of the health facilities in the country. Most senior doctors I had known had migrated to the UK, USA, South America and Japan in search of greener pastures. The young doctors in the system were disgruntled because they were not allowed to leave the country for a few years after their graduation. They also faced shortage of medical supplies. I learnt that most of the medicine and equipment was being imported from India or China. People in the country still depended heavily on the traditional system of medicine, which imbibes a lot from traditional Indian and Chinese medicine. I made it a point to meet the country's health minister and express my concerns. Now, I think the situation is better as The Royal College of Physicians, London, has taken over the post-graduate curriculum in medicine. Hence, I expect that the quality of postgraduate medicine in Burma has gone up.

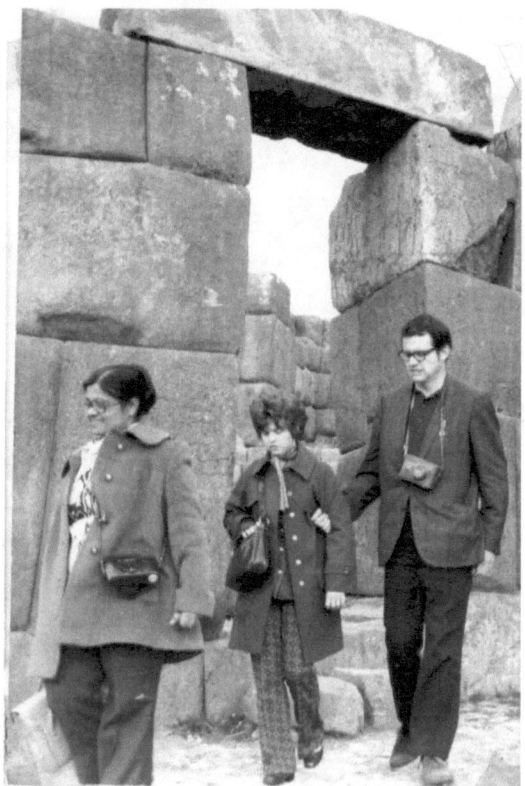

Macchu Picchu

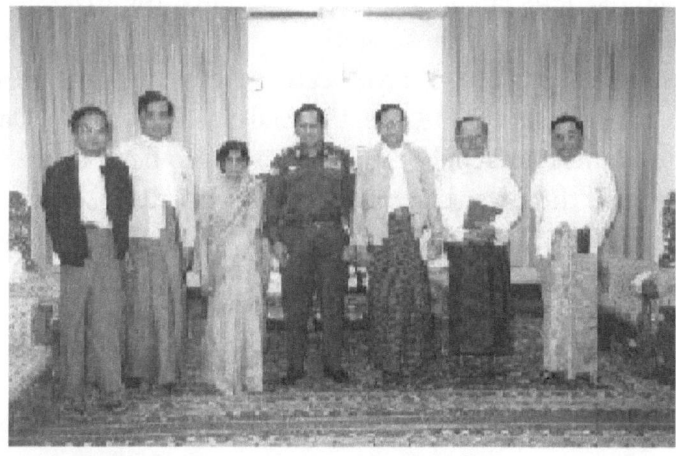

Meeting the Health Minister and Senior Officers at the Secretariat

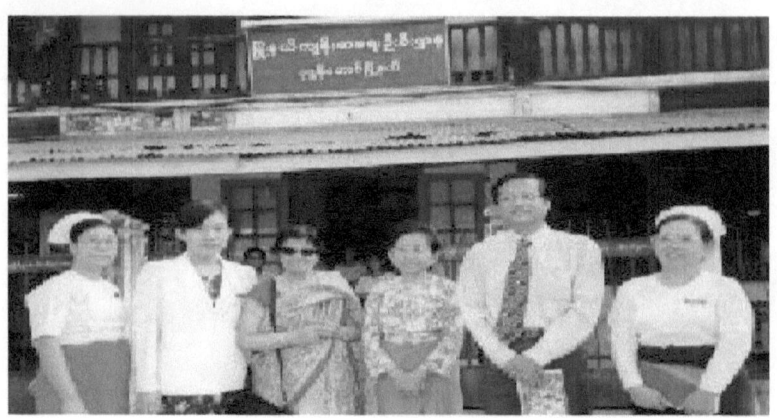

With Burmese Doctor and Nurses

I have also travelled the length and breadth of Israel, planting a sapling on Mount Zion, and making Jewish friends in spite of a sympathy with the Arabs. I have travelled extensively in the Middle East, which I may not be able to do again, visiting Damascus, Baghdad, Lebanon and Syria.

Although it was work that took me to these places, it was my knowledge of communities and cultures also that automatically grew through these visits.

Closer home, in India, I have visited all the states as an examiner for MD and DM exams. These travels allowed me to gradually learn a lot about the similarities and differences in the state of medical facilities across states. I have visited most of India, except for the Andaman & Nicobar Islands. This enabled me to experience the diversity of India. The beaches of some of these states especially Tamil Nadu, Kerala, Goa are breath-taking and I have been there many times. I have also been up in the heights of The Great Himalayas in Bengal (Darjeeling), Uttar Pradesh and Himachal Pradesh. I have also been to the far east of India and visited the seven sisters, enjoying Mizoram, Manipur, Assam, Arunachal Pradesh, Tripura, Meghalaya and Nagaland. They are very different from the rest of India in the way of food, culture, and language.

Bureaucracies and Governments

I formed impressions about bureaucracies in the countries that I visited, but the three that stood out were Russia, the US and India.

Russia

I was invited as a State guest to Russia (then U.S.S.R.) in 1985. We flew by Aeroflot, which was an experience by itself. On landing, I was whisked out of the airport within fifteen minutes, was entrusted to the care of a Lady-in-Waiting, Sonia Buchagova, to take me around the city of Moscow. This included a visit to Leo Tolstoy's house in Ulitsa Lva Tolstog, but I was unable to see his farm in Yasnaya Polyana. I was keen on seeing these places because of my admiration for many of the Russian authors. They evoked so many childhood memories of the books I had read in translation and gave me an insight into the lives of these talented authors.

In my experience, Russian bureaucracy appeared to be the most benign among all the governments I encountered. I do not know whether my impression of the bureaucrats was influenced by my ignorance of the Russian language or the large quantities of vodka which I had to consume every evening. The highlight of the visit was my meeting with Mikhail Gorbachev before the days of Perestroika and Glasnost.

USA

I came face to face with the US bureaucracy because of their equipment donations to my health program on Cor pulmonale. I personally met the Surgeon General of US at the beginning of our association. The officials were very polite and easy going, and did not apply any undue pressure. My interactions and experience with them were always pleasant and my research was not hampered as I received all the equipment in due time.

India

The Indian bureaucracy is the worst, especially the state governments. Officials are rude and without any sense of urgency. They never reply to letters, and when these are received, they are full of obfuscation and signed by officials low down in the scale, indicating that most important matters never even reach the higher authorities. The central government was somewhat better in the days when I dealt with it. It has gotten worse over the years, and nothing can be done these days without greasing palms.

Notable People and Relationships: VIPs and VOPs

Among the many VIPs I have come into contact with, Dr. S. Radhakrishnan, Pandit Jawaharlal Nehru and Mrs. Indira Gandhi are the ones I have immense respect for. My accounts shall focus on these three among the many that I have met, including people of all high ranking categories such as ministers, highly placed bureaucrats, lawyers, and doctors, to mention a few. Though my accounts of Very Ordinary People (VOPs) may not be mentioned in full, they have been the recipients of a large chunk of my efforts and my dedication. I have had significant and varied interactions with people from both these groups throughout my professional life.

I must mention many patients who do not fall into the VIP category but who have formed a significant part of my life, apart from my teachers and school. Gopal Subramanium, eminent lawyer and former solicitor-general, is a grand nephew of mine who has helped me a great deal in tricky situations. Dr. Paul White, who in his lecture at The Fifth World Congress of Cardiology, has said that many patients with heart disease improve with age and that patients seen after hundred years by different doctors have lived a very full life. He has given a list of 86 patients who have lived over a hundred years! Alas, to give a list of my patients whom I have been observing for nearly 50 years would be outside the scope of this book, but I would like to express here my gratitude and satisfaction to them.

VIPs

Dr. S. Radhakrishnan

I had occasion to meet him several times before and during the Fifth World Congress of Cardiology in 1966, which he inaugurated. As a person, he was exemplary, as he put you at ease the minute you met him and was very pragmatic in his approach. I had the privilege of being involved in his treatment in 1967 when he had a stroke and could not preside over the Republic Day Parade. During my visits to Rashtrapati Bhawan, I got to know his son (the historian Dr. Sarvepalli Gopal) and his daughter-in-law, who were a most charming and unassuming couple. I also met him a few times in Madras after his retirement. As he grew older, he suffered from more minor strokes but remained as bright as ever. I consider it one of the greatest privileges of my life to have met him and his family.

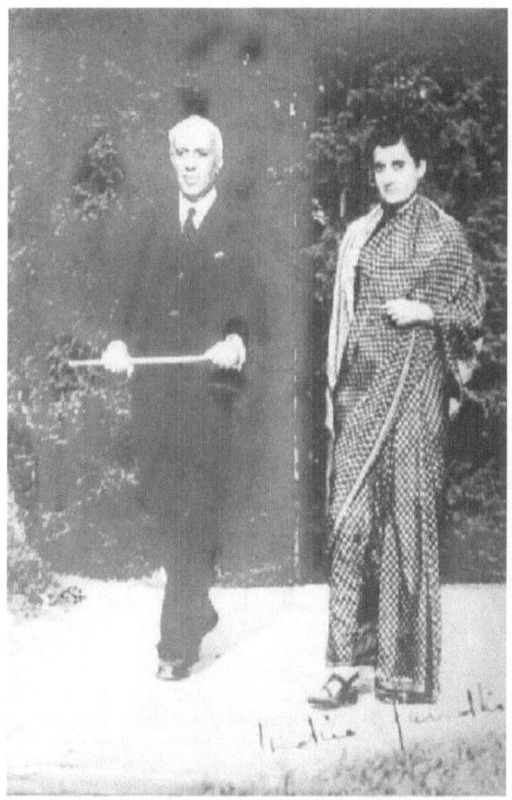

Pandit Jawaharlal Nehru

Incidentally, the first time I met Pandit Jawaharlal Nehru was in April 1937 in Yenangyaung, upper Burma. I quote from an article I had written of tributes to him. He had come there with Indiraji to address the Burmese and Indian labourers in an oilfield town. I was a young student then, and my father—then a leading barrister at Magwe, 32 miles from Yenangyaung—had been invited to the function with his family as he was a leader of the Indian community. Like all expatriate Indians, we regarded India as our real home and had the greatest respect and admiration for our national leaders, with Gandhiji and Panditji heading the list.

I remember being completely awed by him. Indiraji was not very well known at the time. Years later, when I recounted this incident to her, she was amused by it. Panditji made a tremendous impact on the gathering, speaking in Hindi and English. Nationalism was also raising its head in Burma at this time, and as a result, he was received with great enthusiasm. I met him again at Rashtrapati Bhawan in the 1950s, when Rajendra Prasad was President of India. On being introduced, he affectionately put his arm around me and talked very light-heartedly about the LHMC, which is where I was working at the time. His personal charm and easy manners made an indelible impression on me and left me with memories I shall treasure all my life.

Indira Gandhi

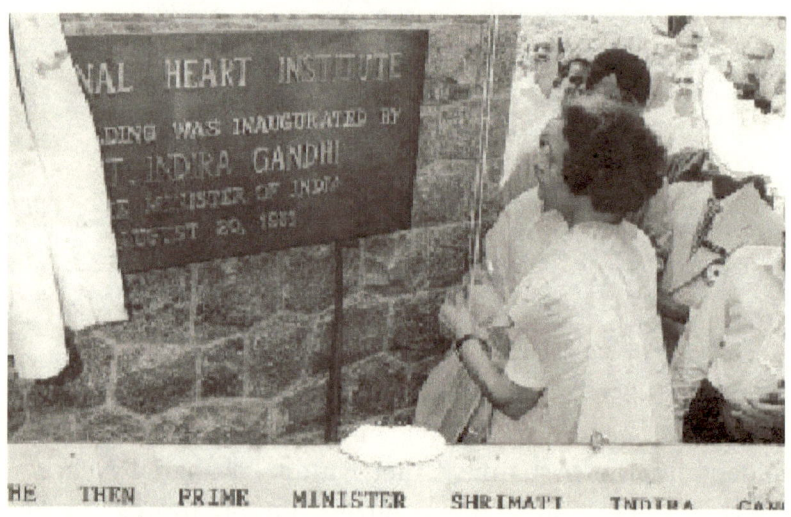

Indira Gandhi Inaugurating NHI

As noted above, my first meeting with Indiraji took place when she visited Burma with her father. Subsequently, I got to know her during several meetings in Delhi at the G.B. Pant Hospital, when she came to visit C. Subramaniam, the Finance Minister; D.P. Dhar, the Planning Minister; and Krishna Menon, the Defence Minister. When I was treating D.P. Dhar during the Simla Summit, I came into regular contact with her and had the chance to get to know her intimately. In August 1981, she very readily agreed to inaugurate the National Heart Institute at my request. She was one of those people whom one gets to like on close acquaintance. I liked and respected her in spite of all the criticism now levelled against her. I was shattered by the news of her assassination.

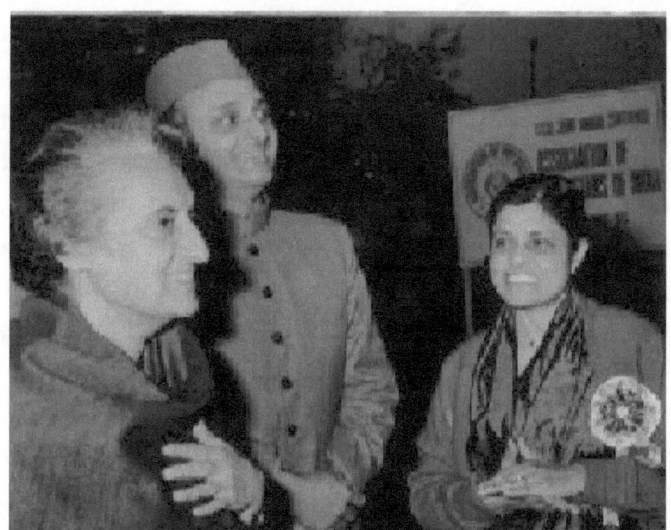

Indiraji Visited MAMC Often

The other VIPs I treated included Mr. Arjun Singh, former Chief Minister of Madhya Pradesh and Minister of Human Resource development, and Raj Narain, former Health Minister of India, and also many others who I do not want to name.

VOPs

Nothing gave me more satisfaction than treating poor patients who could not afford the basic necessities of life. I particularly remember pacemaker patients, whose lives have been extended by over 15 to 20 years due to this device. We first started fitting patients with pacemakers in 1967. I recently met C.L.M., who had undergone 3 pacemaker implantations. He has lived long enough to see his five daughters married! Nearly 300 of my patients to date have been implanted with pacemakers, all of them free. Some of these were rickshaw pullers, vegetable vendors and destitute widows. Among the many lives saved by pacemarkers are:

- Mrs. S., first implanted in 1995 at the age of 21 years.
- Miss. P.K., who has undergone 3 pacemaker implantations. She was first implanted in 1995, then in 2014 and subsequently in 2012.
- Mrs. N.S., having undergone 3 pacemaker implantations, first in 1999, then 2006, and subsequently in 2014.

Of the VOPs that I met, there are a few cases with congenital defects that stand out clearly in my memory. I have followed up with some of these patients with for forty years. One of them was B.A., a woman who came to see me when she was eighteen. She was diagnosed with Eisenmenger syndrome, wherein a two-way shunt in the heart increases pulmonary artery pressure due to mixing of arterial and venous blood. Now fifty-eight, she is married and leads a near-normal life despite having diabetes, which is common in her family.

Another memorable patient is G.T., one who had a congenital heart defect in which the Truncus Arteriosus does not divide properly into what constitutes the artery and pulmonary trunk in a developed human baby at the embryonic stage. I saw this patient when he was five years old. Even though he was not found fit for any surgical intervention as a child, today he is thirty-two, leading a normal life and exhibiting minimal symptoms.

R.L. was another patient with a congenital defect heart whom I treated for the first time when he was eighteen. When he came to me, he had already had a myomectomy and a pacemaker in the abdomen, with the operation having been performed in London in 1974 by Sir Magdi Yacoub, the famous heart surgeon whom I had first met while a postgraduate in Baltimore. I recommended implanting a pacemaker in the abdomen. The surgery was successful, and since then, he has had his pacemaker replaced six times, with good results. He leads a near normal life, at 61.

Tetralogy of Fallot is the most common congenital heart disease. Cyanosis, a bluish discolouration of the skin due to poor circulation or inadequate oxygenation of the blood, is a common symptom, and it is caused due to inadequate blood flow for oxygenation to the lungs. I vividly remember two cases of the many I have seen. These two children were treated with a complete correction in 1973, when they were still infants. They are now both married and have children. One of them came back for a second operation due to complications, which are common and successfully treated.

Of the many RHD patients I have treated over the course of my career, I distinctly remember two who had Bjork Shirley valves implanted in 1983 and are currently in good health.

My Gurus

I have been fortunate to have the guidance of many gurus in my life. I am grateful to my earliest teachers, my father, for instilling in me a love of books and history, and encouraging me to be objective about everything in life, including myself. From my paternal grandmother, I have learnt to be courageous, strong and resilient, and not be hampered by whatever obstacles I may find. I am also thankful to my teachers in school, especially the Englishmen who encouraged my love for literature and mathematics. Later on in life, I was lucky to find medical gurus, who shaped my professional life and personality, much in the same way my teachers in my youth did. Dr. Paul White, Dr. Helen Taussig and Dr. Ancel Keys were the ones who played major roles.

Dr. Paul White

I am proud of having been Paul White's student and having had such a long association with him from my days as a postgraduate. I learnt a lot from him about clinical cardiology and my attitude towards patients. He was also responsible for my forays into international cardiology. There is no doubt that he is one of the greats of cardiology. His wife Ina Reid White was equally lovable, a great friend who I went to see every year in Boston after he passed away. It was due to my studying under him that I contributed to a special edition of the American College of Cardiology in 1962. Below, I have reproduced an account of when Dr. White visited LHMC on May 10, 1961.

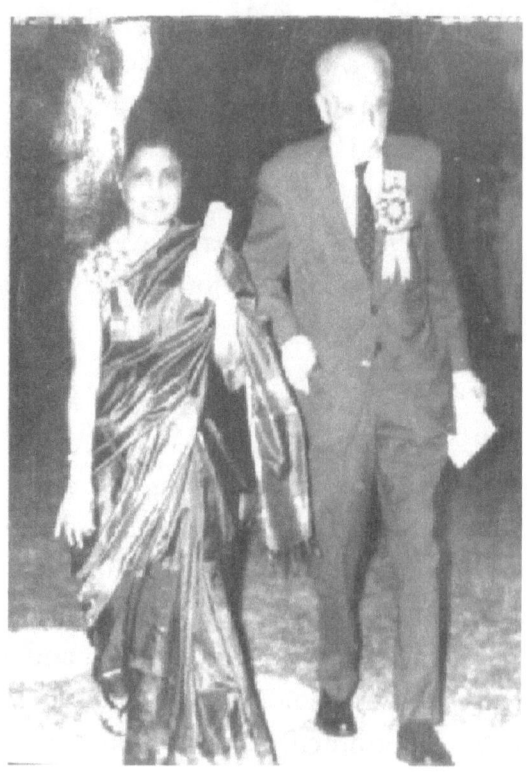

Paul White in India

At 9 o'clock in the morning, there was a gathering of cardiologists, internists and laymen who had come from all over India to meet Dr. White and hear him speak of the need for a cooperative effort to fight heart disease. Prominent among the laymen were patients of Dr. White, who had been easily persuaded to come. Although various types of heart disease account for a large number of lives lost in India, not all present were convinced of the need for such a venture.

Dr. White arrived punctually, even though he had flown in the previous evening from Australia after inaugurating the Heart Foundation in the country and visited the All India Institute of Medical Sciences that morning. He greeted everyone present heartily. There were many that he was meeting for the first time. All of them knew him by reputation but had not expected to find him to be so approachable. There was a free and frank discussion, and it did not take him long to convince them of how successful a joint effort of cardiologists and laymen had been in other countries such as the US, Canada, Finland and now Australia. The meeting ended with unanimous support for the idea of a unified heart foundation in the country.

Within minutes of the meeting, Dr. White was at the Lady Hardinge Medical College, meeting the staff and students and discussing their problems. He had also given appointments to several referred patients. Dr. White made it a point to see each one of them, giving them his undivided attention without haste and taking meticulous notes on small cards he carried with him everywhere. Each patient felt she or he had had all the time he wanted with a man who was extremely busy. He arrived somewhat late for his lunch engagement to meet more new friends and give a long press conference. That was followed by a lecture under the aegis of Delhi University, so heavily packed that there was no standing room. Next came meetings with the Minister for Health and the American Ambassador. At 8 o'clock that night, there was a gala dinner where he gave an illuminating talk. When, around midnight, he said goodbye to the guests, he looked anything but tired, ready to take off for Kabul early next morning. It was at this meeting that Dr. Paul White had sown the seeds for the All India Heart Foundation.

This is a glimpse into the man's visit to India, a country where he is loved and respected. He always made it easy for people to admire him, and I know that he has a similar reputation in many countries. With his extensive knowledge of history, he viewed world problems as one and not as isolated events, and was capable of providing solutions based on scientific knowledge. The added presence of a very sympathetic approach to people further increased my regard for him.

I once asked him the secret to his boundless energy; he smiled and said he took time off now and again to do things he enjoyed, such as chopping wood. I wondered for days if this was really the secret or if Dr. White just had an innate capacity for work and enjoyment of life.

70 | My Life and Medicine

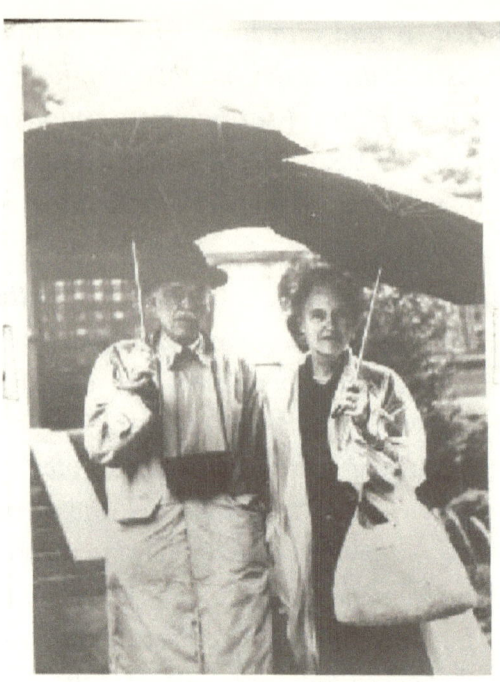

Dr. Paul White and His Wife

Dr. Helen Taussig

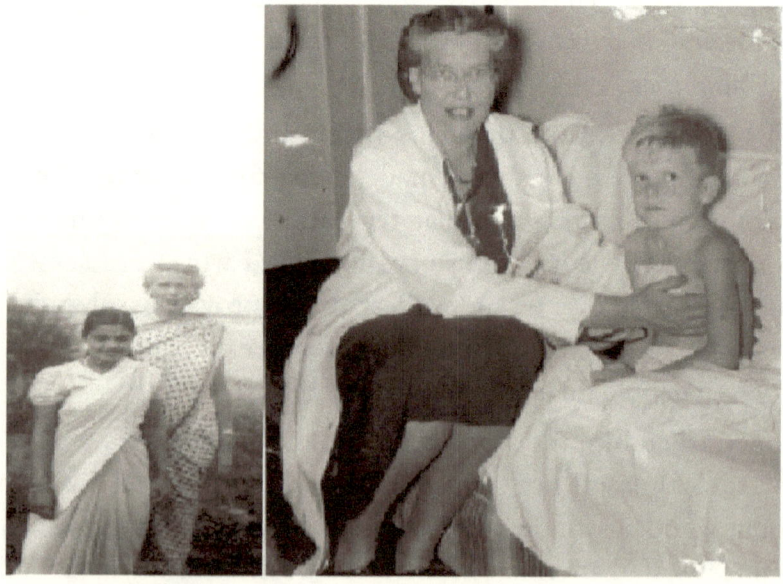

Dr. Taussig   **_Dr. Taussig Examining Baby_**

Helen Taussig was a doctor who was of a different mould. She was affable and very kind to patients, and had remarkable clinical acumen. Technology for congenital heart disease in her time was very limited and confined to clinical examination, ECG and fluoroscopy, but these never deterred her. She is known to have pioneered the use of the X-Ray and fluoroscopy machines for less invasive detection of abnormalities in a baby's heart and lungs.

The doctor was my house guest at LHMC and always interacted enthusiastically with the students and staff. Over the course of my career, she has remained a guru for whom I have the deepest respect and affection. She visited India several times and gave an excellent lecture at the Fifth World Congress. I am very proud to have published with Dr. Taussig the first 1000 cases of Tetralogy of Fallot in the American Journal of Physicians in 1951.

Dr. Ancel Keys

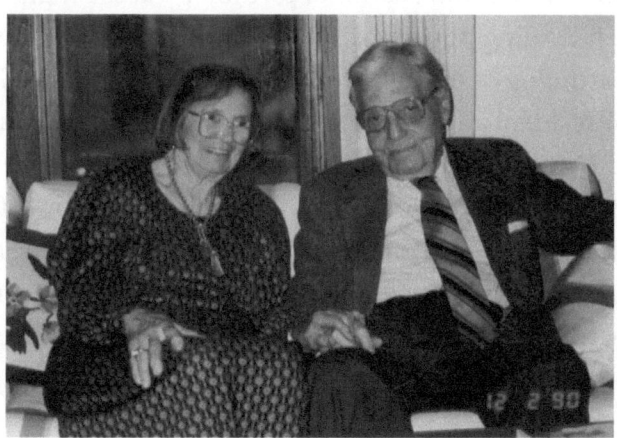

Dr. Ancel Keys with His Wife Margaret

Ancel Keys (1904–2004) and his wife Margaret were great friends of mine. I learnt the basics of cardiovascular epidemiology from Keys, who was responsible for the discovery that dietary saturated fat is a key factor cardiovascular heart disease. His Seven Countries Study revolutionized concepts of ischaemic heart disease and the importance of lifestyle.

He invented two key diets: K-rations, the meals used for soldiers in World War Two, and the heart-healthy Mediterranean diet. His cook book, *The Benevolent Bean*, is a measure of his interest in lifestyle and diet. He authored several other books; *Eat Well and Stay Well* are also on the same lines. *Adventures of A Medical Scientist* was an account of his life and exploits in medicine, which were diverse and many. From these books, I have not only gained invaluable medical insights but also learnt more about Dr. Keys as a person and a professional.

I had the pleasure of also sharing a personal relationship with him and visited him at his clinic in Minnesota and his home at Pioppi, Italy. He has included a brief account of my visit in his memoir. I recollect that time fondly and am honoured to be a part of his splendid research and his recounts.

Positions, Awards and Recognition

I have been involved in International cardiology at the highest levels and have had the following positions. I was a Co-founder of the Asia-Pacific Society of Cardiology (APSC) in 1972, its first Secretary General, and later its Vice President and part of its research committee. I was a member of the World Heath Organization's ad-hoc committee on RF/RHD, and a member of their expert committee on heart disease for fifteen years. I was an overseas member of the Royal College of Physicians, London, for ten years. I was also President of the Asia Pacific Heart Network (APHN), Member, Board of Directors of International Society and Federation of Cardiology, now called the World Heart Federation.

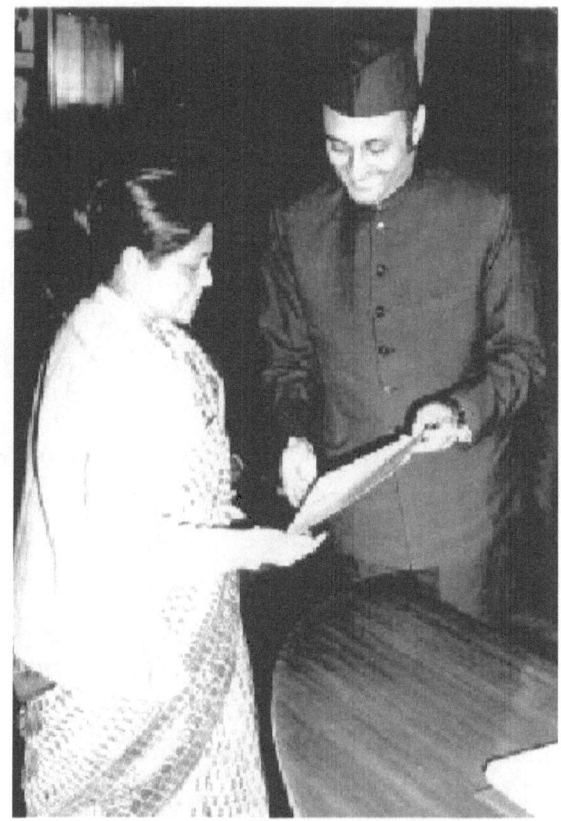

Receiving the B.C. Roy Award

Important positions that I have had the privilege of holding in India were President, National Academy of Medical Sciences, President, Cardiology Society of India, and Member, Research Committee Board of Indian Council of Medical Research. I have been a member of the All India Heart Foundation since 1962 and am its present President. I was also a Member, Board of All India Institute of Medical Science (AIIMS), and Member, Board of the Jaya Deva Institute of Cardiology, Bangalore.

My areas of interest found me involved with multiple research projects and presented the opportunity to attend and organize seminars. For me, garnering experience during my work was the focus throughout my career and also the most rewarding aspect. However, I have also been fortunate enough to receive numerous awards, including the Padma Bhushan (1967) and Padma Vibhushan (1992), without ever applying for any such an honour. My satisfaction has always stemmed from the fact that my seniors and colleagues have thought of me being worthy of these awards. I give below a list of the awards.

- Padma Vibhushan (1992); Padma Bhushan (1967); BC Roy National Award (1975); Harvard Medical International Award (2003); MGR Medical University, Madras – 1991 DSc (Hon.); 1994 Antonio Samia Oration of APSC (2005); S. N. Bhansali Lectureship Award (1967); Tapan Kumar Basu Oration (1969); Lok Bandhu Dr.Bhuvaneshwar Barooah Memorial Oration (1973); Uma Rani Banerjee Memorial Oration (1974); Glaxo Oration (1975); Kamla Menon Research Award (1975); Kamla Puri Sabharwal Memorial Oration (1976); Bhatia Misra Oration, University of Lucknow, Lucknow (1977); Kanishka Award (1977); Devichand Memorial Oration, University of Himachal Pradesh (1978); Bajoria Memorial Oration; Dr. A.K. Chaudhary Memorial Award (1980); Rajaji Ratna Award (1985); K.K. Datey Memorial Oration (1991); Mahila Shiromani Award (1992); Rotary International District 3100 Vocational Award (1995–96); NFI Annual Day Award (1999); Indira Gandhi Priyadarshini Award (2002); Shadak Sharappa Memorial Lecture (2004); FICCI Ladies Organization Award (2005); Sullivan University Eurasia Award (2006); Ph.D. (Hon) Sri Venkateshwara University Tirupati (2008); Sivananda Eminent Citizen Award (Sanatan Dharam Charitable Trust) (2012); Lifetime Award CSI (2012); Lifetime Achievement Award of the National Academy of Medical Sciences (2013); Exceptional Service Award of the Golden Jubilee of G.B. Pant Hospital (2014).

I received the Lifetime Achievement Award (2015) by the Maulana Azad Medical College on their Golden Jubilee day and was guest of honour at the Lady Harding Centenary (founded in 1916) in 2015. I also received a special award by the Deptt of cardiac surgery, G.B.Pant at their Commemoration of 50 years in 2015, and a Distinguished Faculty Award by the G.B. Pant Hospital at their Golden Jubilee National Cardiology update in March, 2015.

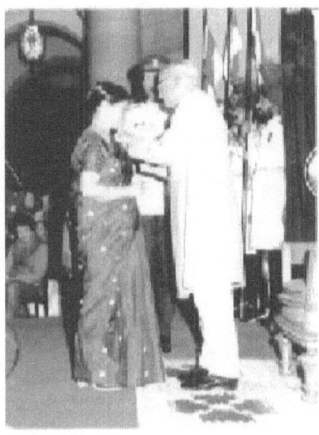

Receiving the Padma Vibhushan (1992)

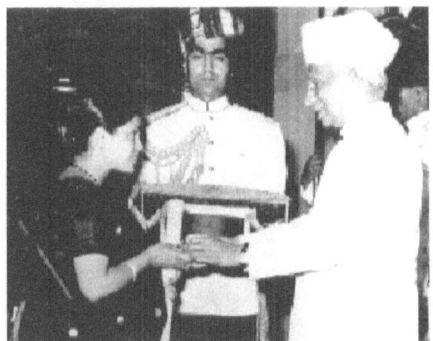

Receiving the Padma Bhushan (1967)

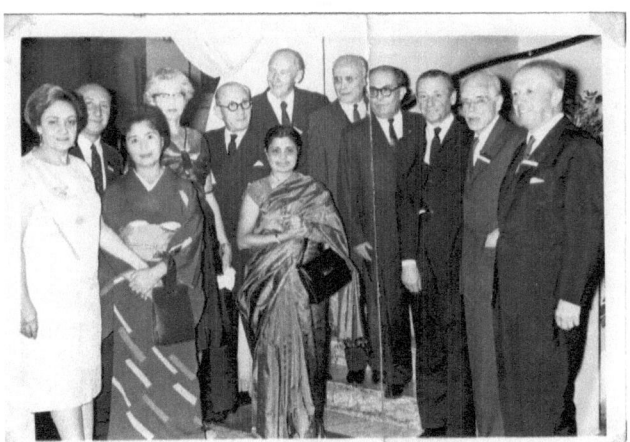

Mexico

Chapter 6
Historical Data and Ancient Systems of Medicine

'For us who believe in physics, the distinction between the past, the present and the future is just an illusion, although persistent'

— **Albert Einstein**

Brief History of Cardiology

Cardiology has had a rich and varied history and has probably witnessed the most rapid growth across medical fields. While its history is a complex subject that can fill several tomes, I will confine myself here to some key developments and highlights.

Although cardiology did not become an independent medical field until about a hundred years ago, even early civilizations were aware of the importance of the heart and heart diseases. In ancient times, when no autopsies or experimental work were carried out, cardiologists relied mostly on symptoms that we now associate with heart disease. Unlike in my experience and that of my colleagues, treatment of these symptoms was largely empirical and experience-based, and successful in many cases. Ancient texts, such as the Egyptian Ebers Papyrus (from 1550 BC), the work of ancient Indian stalwarts Sushruta (~600 BC) and Charaka (~200 BC), the Greeks Hippocrates (460–370 BC) and Galen (130–210), and of the Persian polymath Avicenna or Ibn Sina (980–1037) all record palpitation, swelling of legs and breathlessness as symptoms, for which remedies were successfully suggested in many cases.

Before World War I, there was neither a separate field as cardiology, nor were there cardiologists. Doctors would rely solely on clinical acumen to treat their patients. The few reports on autopsies—such as that of Herrick, who in 1912 showed that heart attacks were caused by blockage of the coronary arteries—revolutionized practices in the field. The tools of cardiology began to appear at the end of the 19th century and early 20th Century. Prominent ones were X-ray machines (1891), the sphygmomanometer for measurement of blood pressure (1881), the polygraph (1902) and the ECG machine (1903). In my own career, I have seen all these apparatus change form, add on features, reduce in size and become far more accurate by leaps and bounds.

Dr. Paul White in *Heart Disease* said that until the late 1940s, there was no treatment for regular heart disease. Antibiotics were ineffective for long-term treatment. He also stated that subacute bacterial endocarditis was always fatal, and that lifelong measures to be adopted after a heart attack were use of a wheelchair and rest. The treatment of high blood pressure was almost a hopeless task. Accounts of the life of President Franklin Roosevelt, who had high blood pressure, corroborate this. The diagnosis and treatment of his heart condition has received a lot of criticism, given that he died of severe hypertension that was not diagnosed properly and not treated, as there were no drugs available for his ailments in those days. The only treatment given to him during World War II was rest and digitalis, and he eventually succumbed to a massive stroke in 1945.

The scenario completely changed after World War II. Before the war, many specialties—including cardiology—were in their infancy. Cardiology was practiced as a special interest by general physicians with superb clinical skills and a few basic tests (ECG, X-ray and some biochemical tests). Coronary artery disease was the most common cause of heart disease in the US by 1910 and in the whole western world by 1950. After World War II, there was great concern for health and related problems as shown by the establishment of landmark organisations linked to cardiac disease.

Vannevar Bush in his book *Modern Arms and Free men* rightly points out that all wars in human history had resulted in improvements in medical diagnosis and treatment. Propagation of advances in mechanical engineering, electronics, hydraulics, sonar and radar can be attributed to the occurrence of World War II. Similarly, the Cold War and moon landings were responsible for important technological developments after 1950. It is now accepted that the phenomenal advances in medical sciences over 1950–2000 far outstrip those in all the previous millennia, and this period is often referred to as 'the 50 golden years'. Hence, it is always relevant to remember that modern cardiology as we know it today developed only recently.

Experience of treating medical problems in all parts of the world and new syndromes, some of which were discovered in concentration camps, all contributed to the development. The International Society of Cardiology (now known as the World Heart Federation, or WHF) was established in 1950 and became a global hub for super specialties, such as cardiology, neurology, nutrition and others. Such super specialties became well-defined fields instead of being areas of special interest of internists. In the UK, the National Health Service (NHS) was formed in 1948 and made medical treatment more inclusive. In the US, the National Heart Lung and Blood Institute (NHLBI) was formed in 1948. The illness and death of President Roosevelt was a key factor in the setting up of the NHLBI along with The Framingham Heart Study by his successor President Harry S. Truman. More than any other societies, NHS and NHLBI were responsible for the development of cardiology due to grants for medical research. In keeping with the post-war momentum, most well-known Western cardiac societies were formed around 1950. In addition to the WHF, NHS, and NHLBI, these included the American College of Cardiology (1949) and the European Society of Cardiology (1950).

In India, the Cardiological Society of India (CSI) was formed in 1948 in Calcutta, with the *Indian Heart Journal* being launched by it soon after. The CSI along with the All India Heart Foundation (AIHF) (1962), the first heart foundation in Asia, created considerable momentum with their annual meetings and research programmes, and are responsible for many of the cardiac developments that we know of today in India. Another key player was the All India Institute of Medical Sciences (AIIMS), which opened in 1956. In 1958, Dr. Sujoy B. Roy, who was born and educated in Burma like me, and also a specialist in RF/RHD, was a professor at Harvard when Rajkumari Amrit Kaur invited him to head up a new cardiology department at AIIMS. India has not lagged behind in starting up institutions dedicated to superspecialties, with the G. B. Pant Hospital (a purely super specialty hospital) being set up in 1964. The Indian College of Cardiology was founded in 1982 and is another key player among cardiac societies.

The research projects led by the funding institutions and societies worldwide resulted in developments at the micro and macro levels of the cardiovascular domain. Cardiovascular epidemiology at the macro level is credited to several Dutch physicians and American physicians working in Indonesia, China and India. As mentioned earlier, Ancel Keys was a key influencer, whose work on The Seven Countries Study expanded the horizons of cardiovascular epidemiology. Such studies have been repeated in several countries with very important results. The first is how lifestyle can influence the development of heart disease, important constituents being diet, smoking and physical activity. At the micro level, isolated heart lung preparation and the study of individual myocytes, mitochondria and genes nudged open the gates of knowledge.

The Human Genome Project (1990–2003) in the US and the UK were two very important research projects that headed the expansion of knowledge in the domain. Apart from a genetics-based approach, molecular approaches were also adopted for micro level studies. All these resulted in better diagnosis and treatment. Advances in genetics, it has been said, are due to twenty particular diseases. Determining genes that are responsible for susceptibility to these diseases is a significant research topic. Genetic causes have been established for diseases such as Wolff-Parkinson-White (WPW) syndrome, long QT syndrome, hypertropic cardiomyopathy (HCM) and familial hypercholesterolemia.

Development of Cardiac Surgery

Cardiac surgery has existed for a very long time, even before anaesthesia become safe. Procedures have evolved at an extremely large scale. Today, the sky is the limit. While it is impossible to provide a history of cardiac surgery in this short space, it is worth singling out a few key developers. Among those who have played a significant role in developing cardiac surgery internationally are C Walton Lillehei, known as the Father of open-heart surgery, as well as Denton Cooley and Donald Ross, among many others. In India, Dr. Reeve Betts started the first cardiothoracic surgery department at Christian Medical College (CMC) in Vellore in 1949. He was joined by Dr. T. Thomas and Dr. N. Gopinath, who started the first open heart surgery programs there in 1960s. By 1975, the first Coronary Artery Bypass Graft (CABG) surgery had been carried out by Dr. K.M. Cherian at Chennai. In 1994, soon after a bill allowing for transplantation of human organs was signed by the President of India, Dr. P. Venugopal and his team successfully performed India's first heart transplant at the All India Institute of Medical Sciences (AIIMS). The patient, Devi Ram, went on to live for another 15 years. In my opinion, cardiac surgery today in trained hands is both safe and effective.

In the field of interventional cardiology, imaging techniques have improved by gargantuan amounts. Apart from X-rays, doctors now have access to CT, MRI and PET, and these are just the most important ones. Among non-invasive techniques, ECHO must be of top priority. From humble beginnings, this technology has now evolved to three-dimensional and four-dimensional ECHO. It has revolutionized the diagnosis of congenital heart disease and many others. Foetal ECHO cardiograph too is a growing subject and key to diagnosis of congenital malformations before birth. This has been used to decide termination of pregnancy or even intra-uterine surgery on the foetus (which is however still in the nascent stages and not practiced routinely at the moment). ECHO has, presently, replaced all other methods of diagnosing congenital defects, making cardiac catheterization an infrequent practice in children.

Rapid progress has been made in investigatory techniques. Before the advances of ECG, which is a late-1970s phenomenon, primitive methods of diagnosis—such as clinical fluoroscopy and later cardiac catheterization in children and adults—were used. Cardiac catheterization was initially carried out in 1929 by Werner Forssmann, who inserted a catheter into a vein of his own forearm and guided it using fluoroscopy into his right atrium. (He lost his job for doing that, but later shared the 1956 Nobel Prize with Andre Cournand for the invention.) By the late 1960's, after popularization by Mason Sones, it became a standard cardiological tool worldwide. In India, the first cardiac catheterisation laboratory for clinical studies was established in AIIMS under the leadership of Dr. Sujay Bijay Roy. Today, catheterization is used to do diagnostic tests such as coronary angiography to detect narrowed or blocked arteries, and to check the pressure and blood flow in the heart's chambers and arteries, to detect heart defects, as well as to extract blood samples and biopsies, and for interventions such as angioplasties with stenting.

All these forms of cardiology are available in developing countries but unfortunately, are not always affordable and accessible for the poor. In my opinion, that is the key aspect in which the medical society really needs to make progress.

Traditional Systems of Medicine

Although allopathic medicine takes pride of place in treatment and education today all over the world, it has not yet found prevention and treatment of all illnesses that afflict the human race. Alternative systems of medicine as they are called are also prominent, although they are old and have not been tested scientifically.

The World Health Organization defines traditional medicine as that "including diverse health practices, approaches, knowledge and beliefs incorporating plant, animal, and/or mineral-based medicines, spiritual therapies, manual techniques and exercises applied singularly or in combination to maintain well-being, as well as to treat, diagnose or prevent illness." It also outlines three types of health systems, in order to denote the degree to which traditional medicine has an impact on the health care in these systems:

The first type is an integrative system, wherein traditional medicine is an official component of all aspects of health care provision (health care delivery, education, training, regulation, and insurance). China, Korea and Vietnam are examples of this system.

The second type of system is the inclusive type. Countries such as the UK, the US, Canada, Norway, Germany, Australia, Nigeria, India, Ghana, Indonesia, Sri Lanka, Japan and the UAE are inclusive systems, in which traditional medicine is acknowledged but not an integral part of the country's health care.

The third type of system is a tolerant one, in which the national health care system is almost entirely based on allopathic medicine, but some traditional medicine practices are allowed by the law. This is the case in Italy.

In the USA, in 1992, US Congress established the office for alternative medicine in the National Institute of Health. The mandate of this Office was extended in 1999, with the Office becoming the National Centre for Complementary and Alternative Medicine (CAM), later renamed as the National Center for Complementary and Integrative Health (NCCIH). It has received progressive budget increases – by 2000, its budget had risen to $68.4 million. Concurrently in 2000, the White House set up the White House Commission on alternative medicine. Created by an executive order on the 8th March 2000, the Commission was charged with developing a set of legislative and administrative recommendations to maximize the benefits of CAM for the general public. It had ten members, including senators and experts, and released its final report in 2002.

The USA also has large number of units for CAM research, based at research institutions such as the University of Maryland, Columbia University in New York, Harvard University in Massachusetts, and the Memorial Sloan-Kettering Cancer Center in New York. International activity in CAM is also becoming more prominent. The European

Union recently completed a COST (European Cooperation in the field of Scientific & Technical Research) project on "unconventional medicine". In 1999, EU Parliamentary Assembly, Member States were called upon to promote to official recognition of CAM in medical faculties to encourage its use in hospitals and to encourage allopathic doctors to study CAM at university level. Also in Europe, the European Agency for the Evaluation of Medicinal Products (EMEA), now renamed to the European Medicines Agency (EMA), works on quality, safety and efficacy of herbal medicinal products. An Ad Hoc Working Group on Herbal Medicinal Products was established by EMEA in 1997.

In India, traditional medicine has been passed down from generation to generation and has become as much a part of the culture as an accepted medical approach. Traditional remedies are commonly adopted for chronic as well as minor conditions and diseases. India is flooded with Ayurvedic, Homeopathic, Unani and Naturopathy products and it is difficult not to use them at some point of time in one's life.

Traditional medicine is holistic. Its success is partly dependent on the user believing in the effectiveness of the therapy. Therefore, the increasing use of these medicine systems can be attributed to the rising dissatisfaction towards allopathic medicine. Today in India, every new hospital has a department dedicated to traditional medicine. These departments outline their treatments on the basis of basic principles of healthy eating, living and meditation. Drugs are prescribed according to the temperament of the person.

In the last century, medicine has indeed evolved, and health care has become more scientific, but the learning of the century before cannot be neglected. Even scientific discoveries have at times stemmed from home remedies. A new book published by the Royal College of Physicians has revealed how plants have contributed to treatment from ancient times. Plants such as the foxglove paved the way for the treatment of dropsy and other plants have been used for the treatment of malaria and blood pressure, to mention just a few. The use of Cinchona has led to the use of Quinine for malaria, the use of Digitalis which was accidentally learnt by William Whithering from an old Shropshire woman who was using it as a cure for dropsy. Other examples are the use of Rauwolfia serpentina, an old Indian drug for high blood pressure, the only one available for many years. Dr. Rustom Vakil introduced it for the western world and was awarded the Laskar award in 1957. The Chinese chemist Tu Youyou discovered how to extract artemisinin for treating malaria, based on a 1,600 year-old recipe entitled *Emergency Prescriptions Kept Up One's Sleeve*, where sweet wormwood (*Artemisia annua*) steeped in cold water was recommended for "intermittent fevers". She received the Nobel Prize in 2015 for her discovery.

Chinese Traditional Medicine

Chinese medicine is one of the oldest in the world. It began around the 8th century B.C. Diagnosis and treatment are based on a holistic view of the patient's symptoms, expressed in terms of the balance of Yin and Yang. Yin represents the earth, cold and femininity. Yang represents the sky, heat and masculinity. The actions of Yin and Yang influence the interactions of the five elements composing the universe: metal, wood, fire, water and earth. Practitioners of Chinese medicine seek to control the levels of Yin and Yang through 12 meridians, which bring energy to the body. Acupuncture, for example, is one of the most widely used Chinese medicine practices is based on meridian theory. It is now practised all over the world. Herbal medicines are also a consistent part of this system. A recent article in *Review of Cardiology* reviewed Chinese medicines said to be effective in many diseases such as high blood pressure, angina and congestive heart failure, however, they state that these drugs need to be tested in a large number of patients.

WHO has set up many laboratories in several countries for testing the efficacy of traditional systems, but it would be true to say that no remedy has been found to be 100% accurate. However, neither disbelief nor total belief in traditional medicines is warranted. There is a lot of scope for research into all these systems as many other remedies have been found effective in small studies.

Arab Medicine (Unani Tibb)

Unani is Greek medicine which developed during the era of Arabic civilization. The name is derived from the Greek 'Ionine', which is called Tibb in Arabic, and is also loosely known as Arabic medicine. It draws from the traditional systems of China, Egypt, India, Persia and the Syrian Arabic Republic. Unani is based on Hippocrates' theory of the four body humours or temperaments: blood, phlegm, yellow bile and black bile. This theory, which also forms the basis for Ayurveda, determines the afflictions of an individual as well as their treatment by particular drugs. The Greek Galen, the Persians Rhazes or Muhammad ibn Zakariya al-Razi (854–925), and Avicenna (or Ibn Sina, mentioned earlier) heavily influenced Unani's foundation and formed its structure. In addition to temperament, the body's natural processes of healing, and particular lifestyle choices are emphasizd. Unani was introduced in India in 1351 by Arabs and flourished under the patronage of Mughals, spreading all over the country. It suffered a setback during British rule but reclaimed its momentum by the endless efforts of the Nizam of Hyderabad and Azizi family of Delhi.

At present the Unani system of medicine has been recognized as one of the Indian systems of medicine and forms an integral part of the national healthcare delivery under the Indian government's Ministry of AYUSH (which stands for Ayurveda, Unani, Siddha and Homeopathy).

Traditional Medicine in India

India today has several systems of ancient medicine in use: Ayurveda and Yoga (63%), Unani (7%), Homeopathy (30%), Siddha (1%). I have already mentioned Unani, so here are overviews of the others:

Ayurveda: Its origin can be dated back to the 10th century BC, but its current form took shape between the 5th century BC. and the 5th century AD, and bears some similarity to the Greek theory of humors. The term 'Ayurveda' is a Sanskrit term meaning the 'science of life', and in fact Ayurveda is not only a system of medicine but also a way of living. The fundamental tenet of Ayurveda is that health relies on a balance between three bodily elements or *doshas* called Vata (air or wind), Pitta (fire or bile) and Kapha (water). Diet, herbs, oil massages, exercise, and lifestyle changes, along with enemas and bloodletting are the tools used to restore health. Ayurveda is widely practiced not only in India but across South Asia in Bangladesh, Nepal, Pakistan and Sri Lanka. Research funded by NCCIH in 2011 found that methotrexate and Ayurvedic treatments for rheumatoid arthritis (based on a combination of 40 herbal compounds) had similar effectiveness. A preliminary clinical trial that year also found that osteoarthritis patients receiving an Ayurvedic compound derived from frankincense gum resin (*Boswellia serrata*) had greater decreases in pain compared to patients receiving a placebo. However, more extensive studies are needed.

Yoga: Yoga ("to join" or "to unite") while now a worldwide practice, has its roots in the Indian subcontinent and has been recorded in the Bhagavad Gita, Upanishads and later in the Yoga Sutras of Patanjali (200 or 400 AD). The purpose of yoga, according to Patanjali, is to still the mind's agitations, and is also described as a kind of "soul therapy". The *asanas*, or exercise postures, make up only one of the eight limbs (*ashtang*a) of yoga practice. In Patanjali's scheme, the second limb is practice of the *yamas*, the Hindu ethical guidelines, with the maintenance of austerities and devotional practices, or *niyamas*, constituting a third limb, and with the remaining five limbs delving into various meditative practices including the well-known forms of breath control known as *pranayama*. Typical modern yoga exercises focus mostly on asanas and pranayama. A recent study in the *European Journal of Preventive Cardiology* reveals that regular yoga practice can result in lowering of heart disease risk through weight loss, lowered blood pressure and lowered LDL cholesterol.

Homeopathy: It was first mentioned by Hippocrates (462– 377 B.C.), but it was a German physician, Hahnemann (1755–1843), who established homeopathy's basic principles, among which the most important is the "Simla Similibus Curentur". The founder wrote that in order to radically heal a certain kind of chronic infection, it is necessary to find remedies which normally cause in the human body a similar disease, as much similar, as possible, Basically, this means that a substance, which absorbed in a certain quantity in a healthy person may cause a disease, may also cure if it is taken in a different dose. Other principles are direction of cure, principles of single remedy, the theory of minimum diluted dose, and the theory of chronic diseases. Homeopathy is widely used in Europe, as well as in Asia and in North America, but so far there has been no scientific evidence supporting it.

Naturopathy and Siddha: An ancient form of traditional medicine, Siddha originated in Tamil Nadu through the work of "siddhars" or scientific saints. Siddha shared many principles with Ayurveda, including the belief in humours, elements and imbalance. Diagnosis involves a key checklist of eight signs and symptoms. Drugs are herb-based and treatments are both internal and external.

The reason for the popularity of traditional medicine is its easy availability and cheapness. India has 6,88,000 doctors and 14,62,000 nurses today according to the Medical Council of India. There are 274 medical colleges in the allopathic (modern) systems, both private (56%) and government (44%), and 400 in the Indian Systems of Medicine and Homeopathy (ISM&H). About 27,000 doctors pass out annually from the modern colleges and a slightly greater number from ISM&H.

How should one deal with the apparent conflict between allopathic and traditional medicine? I believe that both uninformed scepticism and entire belief are wrong. The present perception is that one should keep an open mind on the subject, and although this may sound strange in the present era of evidence-based medicine, many of these remedies may be useful and not harmful. However, some of the medicinal preparations used undoubtedly contain heavy metals which are harmful. Further large-scale scientific studies are definitely needed.

Chapter 7

Heart Disease Today: Global Assessments

Types of Diseases

It is estimated that the number of deaths from cardiovascular diseases (CVD) worldwide will increase to 23.3 million by 2030, remaining the leading cause of death. According to the World Health Organization, in 2015 almost 17.7 million people died of CVDs, constituting 31% of all deaths. Over 75% of these occurred in LMIC (Low and Middle Income Countries), including India. Currently, the world is faced with the following types of CVDs:

Atherosclerotic heart disease, the most common type, comprises disease of the coronary arteries, disease of the brain arteries (cerebrovascular disease) and peripheral artery disease, which affects the arteries of the limbs, kidneys, eyes, etc.

Infectious types of heart disease including rheumatic heart disease (RHD) are still endemic in the developing countries such as India, South Africa, South America and the Middle East, even though they have almost been eliminated in other parts of the world. According to the World Health Organization, there are 25 million persons with RHD in the world today. Bacterial endocarditis, which is inflammation of the heart valves, is another type of infectious heart disease. Viral infections account for a small number but may be related to another condition known as dilated cardiomyopathy (DCM, see below).

Congenital malformations of the heart are another type. It is believed that 10 in every 1000 newborns globally have congenital heart malformations. Many types can be treated with operations today, but surgical intervention can go only so far, leaving a gambit of diseases that cannot be treated.

The fourth type is thromboembolic disorders, which include deep vein thrombosis (clot development within a vein) and pulmonary embolism (clots in the pulmonary artery).

Lastly, there is a group of heart ailments for which causes are not well-known and are still being researched. These are DCM, a condition where the heart muscle or myocardium is abnormal, hypertrophic cardiomyopathy (HCM), where the heart muscle is enlarged, and Kawasaki disease, which results in inflammation of the arteries.

United States

There was a near epidemic of CVD between 1910 and 1965, especially in the 1940s, in people below the age of 65 years. It caused considerable commotion in the population. Since then, however, much research has been done—both at the macro and the micro levels—on the subject and action initiated through research grants largely given out by the National Institute of Health. The basis of CVD was established a long while back, by the work of Herrick in 1912. Since 1967, thanks to the research, there has been a sharp decline of CVD in men.

According to one authority, the era when people dropped dead suddenly is over in the US. It is believed that 40 per cent of the decline is due to better treatment of the actual heart attack and 60 per cent due to control of risk factors. Age and heredity of course are beyond the realm of human control, but other risk factors are all actionable. The risk factor concept was enunciated in 1961 by the Framingham Heart Study, in which age, heredity, diet, physical activity, smoking, high cholesterol levels, high blood pressure and diabetes were held responsible for heart attacks. Control of risk factors has paid rich dividends, especially curbing of smoking and drugs to control high serum cholesterol and high blood pressure. While such controls have been held responsible for the decline of disease in men, in women, however, the picture is somewhat different as they have not been involved in many programs.

Currently, according the 2017 report of the US Center for Disease Control, about 23.4% of deaths in the US in 2014 are due to CVD. However, the US still faces challenges to reducing the number of cardiac deaths further, although the situation is not as alarming and immediate as that in other countries. The epidemic of obesity and diabetes sweeping the world today has also affected the US.

As for RHD, while it was common in the US when I was a student there, it is believed to have died out due to improvements of standards of living and antibiotics.

Europe

While the rate of deaths due to heart conditions has fallen in some countries in the European Union, it is increasing in some others. According to the 2017 report of the European Heart Network, heart disease accounts for 45% of all deaths in Europe as a whole and 37% of all deaths in the part of Europe that constitutes the European Union. Coronary heart disease is the most prevalent cause, and stroke is the second leading factor. In the recent past, the Russian Federation has reported the highest rate of cardiac disease, while France has displayed the lowest. Countries surrounding the Mediterranean Sea usually fall into the group of countries with the lowest rate of heart conditions.

In Europe too, the decline in mortality has been the highest in countries that have shown highest risk factor control. In recent years, the EuroAction programme and Euroaspire programme (co-sponsored by the European Cardiac Society) have had a positive impact. The EuroAction programme has led to government legislation with regard to diet and exercise, and improved ICU care and media awareness has helped. Necessary displaying of nutritional content for all food items, development of better facilities for exercise, such as parks and cycle paths, and prohibition of smoking in public areas have all helped in the decline. Cases of RHD have been noted in Europe since the 17th Century, even when disease was known by different names. It was not until 1868 that the four components (arthritis, carditis, nodules and arrhythmias) were all attributed to one cause. It was a notifiable disease in Denmark and the data of that country testifies to it. As with the US, it is believed to have died out in Europe due to improvements in living standards along with medications.

India

Over six decades, the prevalence of coronary artery disease has increased from 4 to 11 per cent (1960–2010). Rural areas are less affected though rural-urban divide is narrowing. It is worrying that 20 per cent are below 40 years of age. Risk factors are mostly due to existing lifestyle factors—poor diet, low physical activity, diabetes, etc. Hypertension accounts for 19–20% of the cases. Ten cases of congenital heart disease for every thousand live births is also the disturbing statistic in the country. There is a large pocket of RHD, although prevention is advocated and marginally responsible for the decline of the number of patients in some states such as Delhi and Tamil Nadu. RHD cases have reduced to 2 to 4 per 1000 people, but these are still a lot, considering the large population of the country. This disease has been endemic in Indian populations for a while. British military physicians in India before World War II mostly remarked about the rarity of RF/RHD in wards and in autopsies in 1938. However, H. Stott, the first person to study RHD in India seriously stated then that the extent of the problem was identical in India and in London. Publication in Indian journals from 1935 onwards point to high prevalence of RHD in all states of India. It is possible that urban migration around this period, creation of slums, infection caused by overcrowding and perhaps a change in virulence of the streptococcus contributed to this situation.

In spite of many committees being set up, not enough has been done for prevention of heart disease by the government. Some general risk factors, such as a lifestyle that includes a grossly unhealthy diet and that is rife with physical inactivity are of course prominent. Hypertension is one of the major risk factors as well, with 30% of the people in the country suffering from it. However, smoking and hyperlipaedemia (abnormal concentrations of fat in the blood) continue to be less prominent factors than in the West. Thus, 85% of the risk factors are due to the traditional lifestyle and culture in the Indian context. The situation is dire enough to call for a drastic public health intervention by the government.

Chapter 8
Heart Disease in Neglected Groups

For a developing country like India, with aspirations to becoming an economic superpower, the lack of adequate healthcare for hundreds of millions is a glaring and embarassing failing. As the Nobel Laureate Amartya Sen has noted, "neighboring countries like Bangladesh, China and Nepal, with similar or even lower income levels than India, have better health and social indicators, including lower infant and maternal mortality rates…" In this chapter, I will discuss two groups that have been relatively neglected in terms of heart disease treatment.

Women

Women continue to be a neglected group worldwide when it comes to diagnosis and treatment of heart disease. It is only recently that there have been a large number of publications on this subject. Sadly, women usually do not form a significant part of clinical trials, with the result that a decline in heart disease among women has not taken place as significantly since 1979. There has been a call for far more research worldwide on women, a challenge that India needs to take up.

There is a striking difference in presentation of symptoms of heart disease among women and men, with the former more likely to dismiss cardiac symptoms as indigestion in most cases. Symptoms of atypical chest pain are more common in women, as are sudden death, higher morbidity and mortality following coronary artery bypass grafting (CABG) and angioplasty. Risk factors determined so far are the same as in men, such as smoking, high blood pressure, high cholesterol and physical inactivity. However, additional factors include contraceptive pills and hormone replacement therapy.

The average age at which women usually get heart attacks is 10 years more than the age at which men get heart attacks, i.e., after going through menopause. They are therefore exposed to more risk factors and co-morbidities. Women generally show less obstructive and less extensive disease on angiography. Mental depression also plays a larger role in the health of women than in men.

In India, there have been very few publications on heart disease in women. Several studies have flagged multiple risk factors; hypertension dominates the risk, smoking is very rare, and diabetes and physical inactivity are common. Anti-pregnancy pills and hormone replacement therapy are also uncommon factors in patients in India. Rheumatic Heart Disease (RHD) cases among the poor are a substantial target for research, while Balloon Mitral Valvotomy (BMV) remains the largest non-coronary intervention in young and pregnant women.

The *Go Red Program for Women* is a venture that was begun by the American Heart Association, with the support of the World Heart Federation. The objective was to create awareness about heart disease and stroke in women and also prevent it. The All India Heart Foundation has signed a Memorandum of Understanding (MoU) with the World Heart Federation in 2011. A group of women has been formed to raise awareness among the female population about cardiac ailments.

Children

Worldwide, children suffer from the following four types of heart disease: Congenital heart defects (CHD), infectious types of heart diseases, cardiac arrhythmias, and those of unknown origin, such as dilated cardiomyopathy (DCM) and Kawasaki Disease. Of these, the most important are congenital defects and those of infectious origin.

The reported incidences of CHD are 8–10 per 1000 live births. According to a series of research projects in different parts of the world, the rate of occurrence of these incidents has remained constant globally. About one-third of these are critical and require intervention in the first year of life.

There is no community-based data for the incidence of CHD at birth. A large number of births take place at home, mostly unsupervised by a qualified doctor. Hospital statistics are therefore unlikely to be truly representative. Various statistics available for prevalence of CHD show that it varies from 2.25 to 5.2 per 1000 live births. There are a few studies on prevalence of CHD in school children, mainly offshoots of prevalence studies of rheumatic fever (RF) and RHD. These studies are of limited value as a large number of CHD cases are critical and lead to death at a very young age. Approximately 180,000 children are born with CHD each year, nearly 60,000–90,000 of whom require early intervention.

Among infectious heart diseases, RHD accounts for the largest number of cases of infectious heart disease in children in South and East Asia, the Pacific Islands, Latin America and the Caribbean.

As for India, it produces the largest number of children suffering from heart disease in the world! This is partly due to population size, but also because of several other factors that need to be addressed. According to a 2005 publication in the *Indian Journal of Paediatrics*, paediatric cardiac care in India is still in its infancy. The resources are very limited. There are very few specialized paediatric cardiac training programs, and they are concentrated in certain areas of India and are orchestrated through combined adult and paediatric programs. The existing number of trained personnel for paediatric cardiology and cardiac surgery is inadequate. It is only through efforts by NGOs and paediatric societies that Indian standards of paediatric cardiac care can be improved.

Another factor is the prevalence of RF/RHD in India, discussed in Chapters 5 and 7. There have been several research programmes in India aimed at RHD since 1966, ever since the country came to be recognized as a major locus with multiple cases of this cardiac problem. The main emphasis has been on secondary prophylaxis and the Government of

India has selected certain centres for this purpose. It has been shown definitely that one full prophylaxis is obviously desirable, and in fact, some prophylaxis is better than none at all. The duration of prophylaxis has been said to be for lifetime in those with proven RHD, and for 5 years after the last attack in those who have had one attack of RF.

I believe it is instructive to look in more detail at the RHD-related discoveries that my team and I made in work carried out at Lady Hardinge Medical College (LHMC) in Delhi. We were able to show in a school survey over 5 years with 40,000 school children that the control of RF in patients was possible through school health services utilizing doctors and nurses. My team was able to demonstrate that school health surveys, conducted by doctors, were more accurate than those by hospitals and clinics. The reason, we gleaned, was the easy availability of health records of children in schools, under the care of school health teachers and nurses, as opposed to records in unaffordable hospitals that were beyond the reach of most poor patients. Delhi was fortunate to have had regular school health surveys. The only other city to have followed suit efficiently was Madras.

With prior permission from the Health Commission, a study was conducted to understand the pattern of RHD among children. We observed 20,000 students in a study and a control group, each for conclusive results. It was noticed that the number of children infected were effectively less in the control group, when compared with the study group. It remained unfortunate, however, that most cities were unable to carry out similar exercises to diagnose RHD and hence battle it. While these surveys were under way, we did regular check-ups for other conditions such as hearing or optical defects—all viewed as symptoms of RHD—among the students and conducted a number of lectures to equip teachers to identify RHD symptoms.

At LMHC, we gave RHD patients the standard treatment followed in the US and Europe at the time. Firstly, important tests such as an ECG, a throat culture for beta-haemolytic streptococcus, an ASO titre and an ESR were conducted. Next, we kept acute patients under observation until these tests returned normal results and the patients had stabilised.

Chronic RHD patients were injected with six units of benzyl-penicillin every three to four weeks. This stretched over five years to entire lifetimes, depending on signs of heart valve involvements. Those sensitive to penicillin were administered Erythromycin 250 mg, twice a day. Adults, contrary to children, were prescribed orally administered penicillin, given that they were less responsive to injections. However, precautionary measures (such as readily available resuscitation equipment) were always taken while medicating children.

However, today RHD has been put on the back burner in India due to the explosion in CHD, along with the fact that it is a disease that usually afflicts those belonging to the economically weaker section. In my opinion this neglect is very wrong. We need to protect children who are at the beginning of life rather than spend all resources on adult cardiology. RHD remains rampant in most Indian states, while CHD and DCM, in both children and adults are on a steady rise. Balloon valvotomy remains the most important non-coronary intervention. This is usually carried out in young women as patients tend to seek treatment too late for other methods to work. Since surgical costs for all these conditions are unaffordable, the need for donations and the support of agencies such as The Rotary Club become vital.

Cardiac arrhythmia in children poses a separate problem. Except for the use of pacemakers in children, there are no cures. Another form of disease that is not well understood is that of Kawasaki disease and DCM, which may be due to history of viral infection, but this has never been proven.

Facilities for Cardiac Care for Children

There are about fourteen centres in the country that have facilities for paediatric cardiac care, including infant and neonatal cardiac surgery. Of the existing centres of cardiac care, only one is in a government hospital, and the rest are in the private or semi-private sector. The cost of getting treated at one is, therefore, several times higher than in a government hospital. The centres are also very unevenly spaced; most of them are in south India and the National Capital Region. The most populous states, such as Uttar Pradesh, Madhya Pradesh, Bihar, Assam and Orissa, have bare or no resources to treat infants, neonates or children with CHD.

The total number of dedicated paediatric cardiologists and surgeons is also inadequate. The total number of cardiac surgeries for CHD at all cardiac centres is 6,500 per year, of which only one-fourth are for neonates and infants. 98% of infants born with CHD probably do not survive.

The reason for the poor cardiac care is firstly lack of awareness. Most births occur without supervision of a paediatrician. The ability of most paediatricians to detect heart disease is also very limited because of the limited exposure to the subject. There is, therefore, a considerable time lag between diagnosis and referral to a paediatric cardiac centre. The cost of open heart surgery costs in a private hospital is 2–5 times higher than treatment in a government-run hospital, making it unaffordable for a large number of families. Private hospitals excelling in adult cardiac surgery programs discourage paediatric programs as these are more expensive, demanding and associated with higher mortality and morbidity.

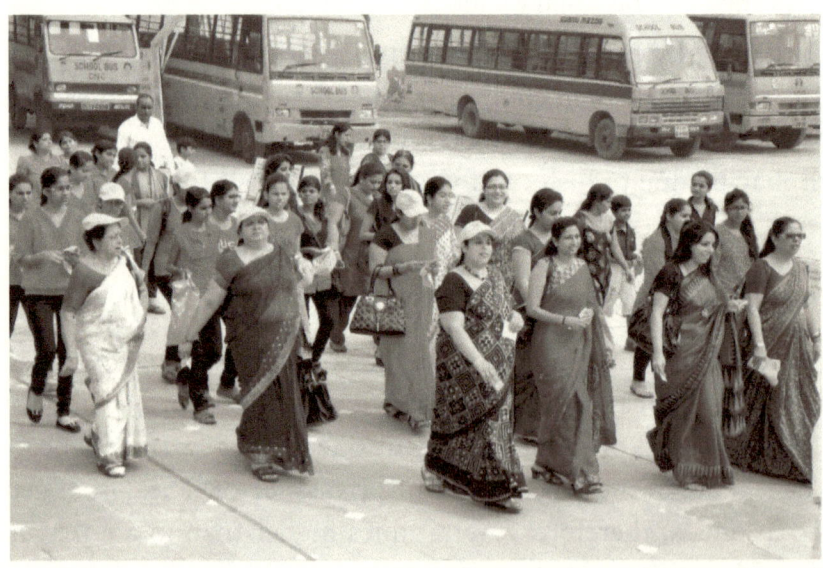

A Go Red Program run by the All India Heart Foundation

Chapter 9

Addressing Healthcare Delivery Gaps through Education

Primary healthcare is provided by the Indian government in most metropolitan cities. There are also a number of super-specialty hospitals and medical centres, but 85% to 90% of these centres fall in metropolitan areas, with around fifty in each major metro city. The rural areas however suffer in acquiring proper health care. The advancements in skill and technology are unfortunately not reaching the poor.

There are many factors responsible for this problem, and addressing it requires both public and private efforts at redressing the inequities. I focus here on education, in terms of providing skilled human resources to address this disparity, as well as increasing public awareness about cardiac health.

Facing up to the Skill Shortage

To ensure more widespread reach and encourage the opening of more such centres across the country, it is essential to involve paramedical personnel in the healthcare delivery system, particularly because of the explosion in technology. Important human resource needs here are nurses, technicians, dieticians and other ancillary workers involved in delivery of healthcare today. Finally, there must be additional incentives for doctors to work in rural areas.

Nurses have been on the scene professionally since the Crimean War. Today, in many countries, there are nurse practitioners who can deputize for doctors. However, the nursing scenario in India is not particularly good, as nurses are poorly paid and do not have avenues for promotion. As a result, there is a large exodus of nurses from India to the Middle East and Western countries, and it is feared that there may be no nurses to man our hospitals in future.

Technology is increasing at a very rapid pace, and special personnel are needed for manning complicated equipment that is widely used today in cardiology. Specialized training programmes are required for technicians involved in non-invasive cardiology procedures—such as ECG and ECHO technicians, nuclear cardiology technicians and radiology technicians. For the operation of heart-lung machines, perfusionists are essential. Technicians involved in cardio-pulmonary perfusion are usually trained at the manufacturing companies itself, and many of them can be very helpful in assisting and conducting some of the work of doctors, who would otherwise spend their valuable time on equipment. Medical centres also require many more physiotherapists and dieticians. Health assistants constitute another important category and play extensive roles in eldercare and hospice programs in the US, Australia, etc. Such professionals can play a major role in India, and this sector needs to be developed much further.

Given the high level of heart disease in a country with more than 1.3 billion people, we need thousands of cardiology-savvy doctors to be produced each year. Cardiologists in India generally have an MD specializing in Cardiology and only hundreds are trained each year. After getting their MD, they prefer to work in big cities where the earnings are higher. However, doctors whose main degree is only an MBBS are likely to be more flexible about working in underserved populations in small towns and rural areas. Training the latter with postgraduate cardiology diplomas is an excellent way of helping address the gaps in cardiology services outside the metro areas.

Human Resource Development at AIHF

The All India Heart Foundation (AIHF) has always endeavoured to train more human resources to meet the severe shortage of paramedics and nursing staff in the country. Nurses are trained in cardiac nursing through short-term courses, and courses in dietetics, nutrition and ECHO have also been carried out. In a recent survey, some points came to light. Earlier, most nurses were being recruited from Kerala. Most of them were Christian and female. Today, we have 101 nurses, and among them, 27 are male. Both male and female nurses in AIHF are from different sections and states in the country. Among the men, 19 are Christian, 7 Hindu and one Buddhist. Of the women, 40 are Christians, 23 Hindus, 5 Buddhists, and 6 Muslims. 29 nurses hail from states other than Kerala. 16 are from Manipur, 5 from Tibet and 8 from Uttar Pradesh. The fact that they come from many different states shows that the society is more open to the idea of medical services, and it is no longer stigmatized. All regions and religions, as well as different social classes, are now taking to nursing. It is a good trend. We must discard the old beliefs and practices that come with treating these services and jobs unfit for any section.

Training in cardiology is provided through the D.N.B. (Cardiology) degree from the National Board of Medical Exams in Cardiology. There is also provision for staff to do a Postgraduate Diploma in Clinical Cardiology (PGDCC) with Indira Gandhi National Open University (IGNOU) and a Postgraduate Diploma in Preventive Cardiology (PGDPC) via Jamia Hamdard. In addition, AIHF has also provided training to physiotherapists, dieticians, and ECG and ECHO technicians.

This data on addressing skill shortages pertains to the late 20th and early 21st Centuries, and thankfully, the situation is continuing to improve.

Public Education: Role of Cardiac Societies

Cardiac societies in many countries have played an important part in the training and treatment of the underprivileged. In India, there are three important cardiac societies today—The Cardiac Society of India (CSI), The Indian College of Cardiology and the All India Heart Foundation. The first two deal with technical problems of cardiology, hold regular annual meetings and have a large attendance, while the AIHF is an important addition with both laymen and doctors as members. The organization also works closely with the CSI, and doctors of the AIHF are also members with the Indian College of Cardiology and CSI.

Foundations are more accessible to patients, involving lay people as well. The very successful ones are the American Heart Association (which is both a society and a foundation), the American College of Cardiology (which has both components), the British Heart Foundation (which has established thirteen professorships in the UK), the Cardiac Foundation of Australia and New Zealand, and the Japan foundation. Next in line are the Heart Foundations of Malaysia and perhaps of India, which are both very active and not limited to one area.

The AIHF's main objectives are public health education in matters of cardiovascular disease and their prevention, research to improve diagnostic and therapeutic modalities, training of cardiac personnel of all types, and population outreach to increase awareness among people below the poverty line through free heart care, pacemakers, ICDs, heart valves, etc. It has achieved all this by its golden jubilee, but there is always scope to expand each of these activities.

With growing literacy in certain sectors of the population, written materials have an important role to play. The AIHF has consistently published its own newsletter every quarter since 1963. A book on heart disease for readers without medical backgrounds has been published in English and translated into Hindi, Marathi, Urdu, Sindhi, Tamil, Punjabi and Kannada. Radio talks, TV interviews and lectures on various aspects of heart disease are regular initiatives undertaken by the foundation. Special days have been observed for creating awareness about diabetes (November 14) and consumption of tobacco (May 31). World Heart Day (September 29) is observed by many hospitals, and sessions with the general public and a walkathon are special features of this programme.

Population outreach has been very important part of the activity of the Foundation. Heart camps are held at least twelve times in a yearin different locations to create awareness. Free check-ups are conducted for a large number of patients and these people are then encouraged to have annual check-ups. Videos on smoking, diet and exercise are shown, and talks are given on many aspects of heart disease, especially prevention. The latest is the Go Red programme for women.

Another programme in the works is for children, involving monitoring blood pressure and determining prevalence of heart disease. Ministers are usually involved in these activities to increase awareness. A special feature is a donation of free Pacemakers and ICDs to poor patients, especially those who are below the poverty line. This has been done since 1988, and over the years, patients have been able to prolong their lives by even up to 20 years in many instances.

Chapter 10

Preventive Cardiology

An age-old adage says 'an ounce of prevention is worth a pound of cure', and these words are to be boldly marked when it comes to heart disease. Treatment of heart diseases is expensive and time consuming. Prevention is not only far easier, but also often more beneficial. It is particularly pertinent for people who belong to the economically weaker sections, as medical assistance in hospitals and cardiac centres is expensive. To adequately address prevention requires a joint effort between the government and the private and non-profit healthcare sectors. As Dr. Paul White emphasized, "The first priority in all our health activity must be that of prevention, and for this doctors need as partners lay industry and the Government."

The good news is that many cardiac patients improve with age, outgrow their troubles, often serious, either spontaneously or with medical and surgical help. Some of them are actually better at 60 than they were at 50, or even at 70 than they were at 60. This fact we did not know years ago. Of course, the reverse case of declining health due to heart disease is unfortunately often true, but the virtues of optimism and patience, along with medical and surgical therapy, need to be cultivated assiduously in every case.

Heart disease of many kinds is certainly more common in India, but even more common, many times over, is the fear of heart disease. This fear is the result of several factors often in combination. First, heart disease is a popular topic in the media and in social gatherings. Second, heart disease is often mimicked by symptoms due to other troubles such as indigestion, sometimes called 'cardio spasm', or a syndrome related to anxiety called neurocirculatory asthenia, not to mention severe anaemia and other prostrating conditions. Third, misinterpretation of electrocardiograms is very common in India, including an over-emphasis on minor or relatively minor abnormalities.

People suffering from heart disease can be followed for years with annual examinations unless some additional trouble develops. There is very often no need to change one's way of life except to get rid of bad health habits like physical indolence, obesity, alcohol, and tobacco. The risk factors are mostly traditional (improper diet, low physical activity, smoking, diabetes, hypertension), and are all preventable.

Sadly, the state of heart disease prevention in India as whole is woeful. Primary care is practically non-existent. Tertiary care is inaccessible to the majority. Insurance is elementary. There is no action by the Government by way of legislation with regard to packaged foods, provision of bicycle paths, open spaces, etc. Smoking has been made at best a timid entry. The media and the NGOs need to step up their efforts considerably.

Prevention Strategies

Three are three types of prevention programmes —primordial, primary and secondary. Primordial prevention has everything to do with prevention of appearance of risk-enhancing symptoms and involves a general guide to the population to curb the risk of heart disease.

Primary prevention is prevention of risk factors. It requires that awareness be created, which is being carried out by several bodies these days.Observance of World Heart Day (September 29) has gone on for 18 years, ever since it was declared by the World Heart Federation under the inspiration of the Spanish cardiologist Dr. Antoni Bayés de Luna, and it has gradually helped improve awareness of heart disease and its prevention. Less well-recognized are World No Tobacco Day (May 31), and World Diabetes Day (November 14). Newspapers, media, TV and radio have all joined to observe these demarcated events through walkathons and large-scale participation. Celebrities and politicians giving a briefing on these topics is also a trend that has caught up in

India now. Regular check-ups at specialized centres are catching on and being increasingly promoted.

Secondary prevention is necessary in high-risk cases, in patients after heart attack, as well as those with a family history of risk factors, including inappropriate diet, obesity, lack of exercise, diabetes, high blood pressure, and high blood lipids. Secondary prevention is well established, better than other types of prevention.

Before beginning a preventive programme, quantification of risk should be carried out. Several important methods of risk calculation have been developed and are in practice today. Current strategies have been based on the quantification of absolute short-term (10-year) risk, as well as strategies of lifetime control of risk factors. A recent type of risk quantification is by the amount of calcium in the arteries, which is much simpler and more accurate than others.

My overall recommendation for prevention of chronic disease is a fairly obvious Six-Point Guideline based on age-old wisdom, and can be summarized in *Table I*.

Table I – Six-point Guideline for Prevention of Chronic Diseases

1. Eat wisely
2. Exercise regularly
3. Watch your weight
4. Don't smoke or use chewing tobacco in any form
5. Restrict alcohol
6. Have a regular check-up for blood pressure, blood sugar, and lipids

Let me now turn to specific risk factors for heart disease.

Specific Risk Factors

1. Smoking and Tobacco Use

Legislation to restrict smoking by raising taxes is extremely important. This is being done in the industrialized world with good effect. Forbidding the sale of cigarettes to those under 21 and the absence of tobacco vendors in the vicinity of schools are other measures that have been taken. Prevention of smoking in public places such as schools, hospitals, cinemas, airplanes is rightly mandatory. Warnings on cigarette packs also help curb the sale of cigarettes. The recent phenomenon of using e-cigarettes is also not free of nicotine, but it does lead to lower consumption. Although it is not ideal, it is a step in the right direction. Professional support and no smoking clinics are a must for preventing smoking. Nicotine replacement therapy, the use of drugs such as varenicline should be offered in no smoking clinics. Other types of tobacco used are equally noxious. This includes chewing tobacco in all forms, including snuff and varieties of *paan* laced with tobacco or nicotine like *gutka, khaini,* etc. Non-smoking tobacco has been shown to cause cancer of the mouth, upper respiratory tract, oesophagus, and stomach.

2. Blood Pressure

A regular check-up once a year is recommended to monitor blood pressure, blood glucose and blood lipids. Hypertension is suspected when office blood pressure is above 140/90. ABP monitoring is recommended to confirm the diagnosis of high blood pressure if daytime mean high blood pressure is more than 135/85. People with an office blood pressure of more than 160/100 in a 24-hour should be offered pharmacological therapy. Others should be given treatment according to established guidelines with drugs such as ACE (angiotensin-converting enzyme) inhibitors, ARB (angiotensin-receptor blocker) as initial therapy or CCB (calcium channel blocker).

3. Diabetes

For Type II Diabetes, glycaemic control is important. The aim should be to maintain HbA1c (glycohaemoglobin) of below 6, fasting blood sugar < 110mg/dl. Also, a professional lifestyle approach is advised for patients above 40 years, irrespective of cholesterol values. Fibrates (fibric acid derivatives to lower blood triglyceride levels) should not be prescribed.

4. Blood Lipids

Non-fasting blood samples should be taken to measure total cholesterol. Statins (drugs to lower cholesterol) are recommended as they are highly effective. The aim is to lower total cholesterol, LDL (or 'bad') cholesterol and triglycerides, and raise HDL (or 'good') cholesterol. For annual checkups, it is fine to do basic tests—such as ECG, ECHO and TMT (Treadmill Stress Test)—and intensive tests are not necessary. Cholesterol-lowering drug therapy is recommended in all patients with established CVD, individuals at high risk of CVD, those who have diabetes and are over 40, and people who have chronic kidney disease.

Pharmacological therapy includes the use of drugs for high blood pressure when needed for blood lipids and for diabetes. An important invention in the field of cardiology has been the poly pill, which contains aspirin, an ACE inhibitor and beta blocker, and an anti-diabetic drug.

Table II indicates some of the ideal results from a health checkup.

Table II – Ideal Health Check Results

Body Weight	Keep BMI 18.5 to 24.0
Blood Pressure	< 140/90 mmHg
Blood Sugar (glucose)	< 110 mg/100 ml (Random)
Serum Cholesterol	< 200 mg/100 ml
Serum Triglycerides	< 130 mg/100 ml
Lipid Profile	High HDL, Low LDL

5. Diet

The key dietary recommendations for heart health are shown in *Table III*.

Table III – Dietary Guidelines

Carbohydrates	Use Complex Carbohydrates
Fats	< 30% of Total Calories (10% Saturated, 20% Poly Unsaturated)
Fibre	In abundance
Protein	Use vegetable sources and Lean Meat, Chicken, Fish, Skim Milk Products
Salt	6 gms/day
Smoking	No smoking the norm and No chewing tobacco
Alcohol	Restrict to few days in the week, not more than 30 gms/day

The well-known Food Pyramid is shown in *Figure 1*.

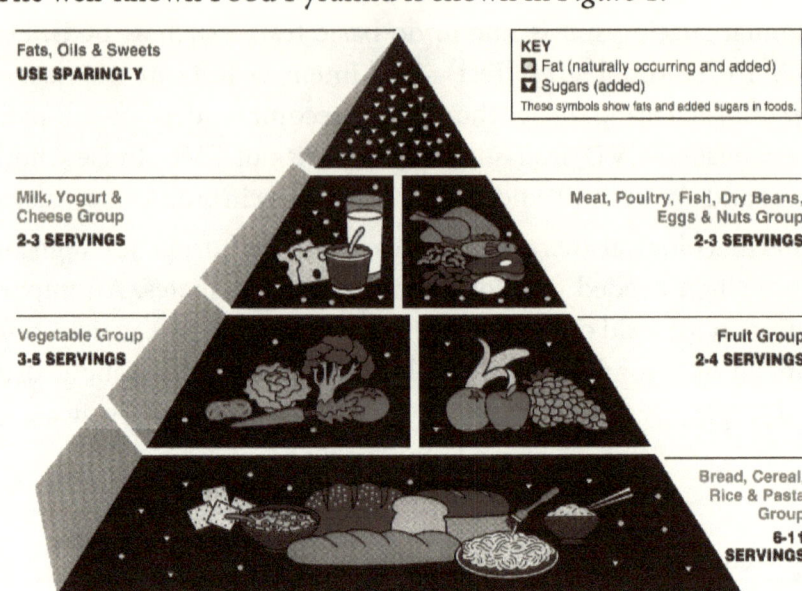

Figure 1: The Food Pyramid

6. Obesity and Weight Control

Monitoring the body mass index (BMI) is an important factor in determining a person's health. *Table IV* illustrates the specific classifications of obesity based on BMI.

Table IV – Classification of Obesity by BMI

Obesity Class	Caucasians	Asians
Under-weight	< 18.5	< 18.5
Normal	18.5–24.9	18.5–23
Overweight	25–29.9	23–27.5
Obesity I	30–34.9	27.5–32.4
II	35–39.9	32.4–37.4
Extreme obesity III	> 40	> 40

7. Exercise

Physical activity goes hand in hand with diet to prevent heart disease. It should be tailored to include at least 30 minutes of exercise per day in addition to domestic chores. Prolonged sedentary behaviour should be strictly avoided.

Unfortunately, all types of house work and daily activities do not amount to enough physical activity to keep heart disease at bay. The pulse rate should be increased to above 70 per minute for at least 30 minutes every day. Exercise or training for at least 150 minutes per week in bouts of more than 10 minutes takes care of this requirement, or alternatively, 75 minutes of rigorous physical activity is advised. One has to keep in mind, however, that warm up and cool down are important components of exercise. Activities that constitute light physical activity are hiking, gardening, bicycling (more than 10 miles per hour), and weight training (general light workout). Vigorous training includes running or jogging at 5 miles per hour, bicycling (more than 10 miles per hour), swimming (freestyle laps), aerobics, brisk walking (4½ miles per hour), weight lifting and basketball.

Prevention of Congenital Heart Disease

Of the known risk factors, Rubella or German measles has been proved to be associated with a large number of congenital defects. Exposure to German measles in young girls used to be a favourite method of prevention. A vaccine for German measles is available and should be used in high-risk cases. In-vitro diagnosis of congenital defects is possible today with foetal ECG, imaging and echocardiography. Foetal surgery has been carried out in a small number of infants in-vitro, but it is not yet a standard method. In the case of defects not compatible with life, abortion is a well-known method. This is already happening in cases wherein Down's Syndrome is diagnosed after foetal ECHO. In the future, modification of parents' genes may also be possible.

Prevention of Rheumatic Heart Disease

Rheumatic Heart Disease (RHD), which I discussed in Chapters 5, 7 and 8, has been one of my abiding interests, and still intrigues me to this day. Prevention of RHD still follows the same methods as used in Europe and the US since the 1950s because these countries have lost interest due to the decline in the disease.

Primary Prevention of RHD

Today, primary prevention has been largely concentrated on the development of the rheumatic fever vaccine to be given in endemic areas. This has been difficult because of the larger number of strains involved and other problems. If a programme fructifies, it will be similar in scope to vaccines given at present for diphtheria, smallpox, measles, etc.

Methods of primary prevention involve injection of the most effective drug for prophylaxis, i.e., benzethene penicillin. It has been recommended that registries of RHD be set up in all medical colleges with departments of cardiology or medicine. Their goal is yet to be achieved. In the 21st Century, wherein coronary artery disease threatens to engulf developing countries, RHD should be eliminated so that resources are not totally diverted from children to adults.

Table V illustrates the present methods of primary RHD prevention.

Table V – Primary Prevention of Rheumatic Heart Disease

Agent	Dose	Mode	Duration	Rating
Penicillins				
Penicillin V	Children: 250 mg 2–3 times daily <27 kg Adults: 500 mg 2–3 times daily	Oral	10 days	IB
Amoxycillin	50 mg/kg once daily (max 1 gm)	Oral	10 days	IB
Benzathine penicillin G	600,000 U for < 27 kg; 1,200,000 U for > 27 kg	Intramuscular	Once	IB

	For individuals allergic to penicillins			
Narrow spectrum cephalosporin (Cephalexin, Cefadroxil)	Variable	Oral	10 days	IB
Clindamycin	20 mg/kg/day in 3 doses (max 1.8g/day)	Oral	10 days	IIaB
Azithromycin	12 mg/kg once daily (max 500 mg)	Oral	5 days	IIaB
Clarithromycin	15mg/kg/day divided BID (max 250 mg BID)	Oral	10 days	IIaB

Secondary Prevention of RHD

Secondary prevention of RHD consists of early identification in children, preferably primary school children and continuous prophylaxis, mostly with penicillin by injection or tablets up to the age of 25 or more. Surgical treatment comes later and is really a last-minute effort to control the disease. It is certainly easier than primary prevention.

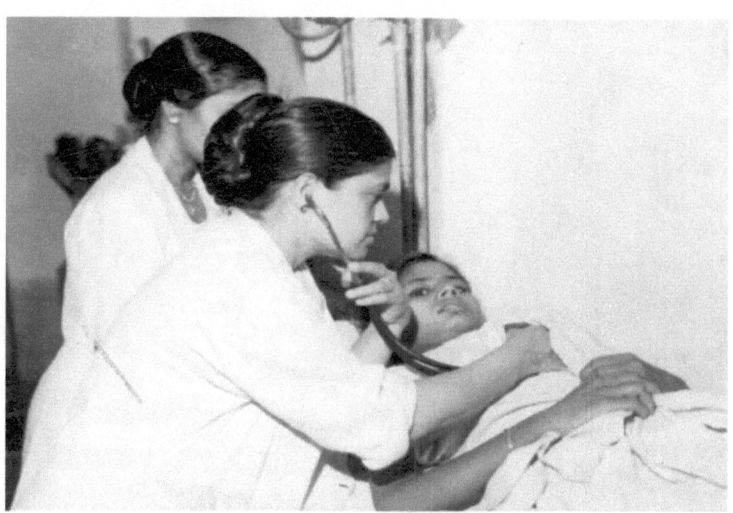

Epilogue

I write this last part with much hesitation. If development, techniques and treatment are to be judged by recent reports, cardiac diseases are likely to almost disappear.

Humans have been improving their lifespans for over 5,000 years. The World Health Organization defined life expectancy as the average number of years a person is expected to live on the basis of current mortality rates. In India, it used to be around 42 in 1960, and it steadily climbed to 62 in 2000. From the standpoint of cardiology, I can do no better than to reiterate the three points made by my Guru Dr. Paul White:

First, we should begin preventive measures against Athersclerosis and thrombo-embolism before we have 100 per cent of the proof of their effect to those of us who have followed the scene for half a century. We know enough to begin the three measures which are very sensible – the avoidance of over-nutrition, the establishment of physical fitness, and no tobacco. Second, we may some day discover magical therapy, but until we do, we have enough to do to protect us and third, I am optimistic about the future in view of our achievements of the past and our present zeal in the prevention of disease. Let us get on with the job.

There is no doubt that congenital heart disease will be contained by gene therapy injections, preventive vaccinations and foetal echocardiography. There is also hope to contain infectious heart diseases through new therapeutic regimens. Coronary artery disease, the main killer today, may also be able to be controlled through simple remedies, as it is believed to be a multi factorial disease, including use of the poly pill.

It is possible that we will have a generation envisaged by the playwright George Bernard Shaw in *Back to Methuselah*. Life will be prolonged and free of disease. I will leave my readers with this thought and hope that developing countries with impoverished populations will have the benefit of the accumulated knowledge, that prevention will be the order of the day and the need for treatment will be minimal.

Bibliography

General

1. Shway Yoe. The Burman: His Life and Notions. Macmillan and Co., 1935.
2. Nehru: The Nation Remembers: Tributes from the members of the national committee for the commemoration of the Jawaharlal Nehru centenary. 14th Nov., 1989.
3. G. E. Harvey. History of Burma. Longman, Green and Co., 1935.
4. Louis Allen. Burma, The Longest War, 1941–1945. Palgrave Macmillan, 1984.
5. George Orwell. Burmese Days. Harper and Bros., 1934.
6. Amitav Ghosh. Exodus from Burma, 1941: A Personal Account, Parts 1, 2 & 3. http://amitavghosh.com/blog/?p=432.

Medical References

Cor Pulmonale

1. Padmavati S, Pathak SN. Chronic Cor Pulmonale in Delhi. Circulation XX (3), September 1959, pp. 343–352.
2. Padmavati S, Joshi B. Incidence & Etiology of Chronic Cor Pulmonale in Delhi. A necropsy study. Diseases of the chest 64 (4), October 1964. 99, pp. 457–463.

3. Padmavati S., Raizada Veena. Electrocardiogram in chronic Cor Pulmonale in Delhi. British Heart Journal XXXIV (7), pp. 658–667.
4. Padmavati S., Raizada Veena. Cardiac Arrhythmias in Chronic Cor Pulmonale. Indian Heart Journal 27 (3), pp. 49–54.
5. Padmavati S., Raizada Veena. Haemodynamics in Chronic Cor Pulmonale. India Heart Journal 27 (2), 1974.
6. Padmavati S. Arora R. Sex Differences in Chronic Cor Pulmonale in Delhi. British Journal Diseases Chest 1976, 70, pp. 251–59.

Rheumatic Heart Disease

1. Padmavati S. Epidemiology of Cardiovascular Disease in India. Circulation, Vol. XXV, April 62, pp. 703–710.
2. Padmavati S., Datey KK. Epidemiology of Cardiovascular Disease in India. M. Eliakim & H. N. Neufield (Eds.) Cardiology current Topics & Progress, Academic Press 1970, pp. 50–53, 1970.
3. Padmavati S. Rheumatic fever & rheumatic heart disease in developing countries. Bulletin of the World Health Organsiation. 56 (4), pp. 543–550 (1978).
4. Padmavati S., Shreshk NK. Prevalence of Rheumatic Heart Disease in Delhi School Chidlren. Indian Journal Med. Res. 69 May 1979, pp. 821–833.
5. Padmavati S. Community Control of Rheumatic Heart Disease in Developing Countries: 2 Strategies for Prevention & Control. WHO Chronicle 34, pp. 389–395 (1980).
6. Strasser T, Dondog N, KholyEL K, Charagogloor, Padmavati S, Kalbian VV, Ogumbi O, Stuart K, Dowd E & Bekery. The Community Control of Rheumatic Fever & Rheumatic Heart Disease. Report of a WHO International Cooperative Project. Bulletin of the World Health Organisation 59 (2), pp. 285–294 (1981).
7. Padmavati S, Rheumatic Fever & Rheumatic Heart Disease in India. Chapter in Progress in cardiology: Leg & Febiger: Vol. XV 1987, pp. 169–183.

8. Padmavati S, Gupte Vijay, Prakash Kunti, Sharma KB. Penicillin for Rheumatic Fever Prophylaxis-3 Weekly or 4 weekly schedule? Journal of Association of Physicians of India. Nov 1987, Vol. 35, pp. 753–755.
9. Padmavati S, Gupte Vijay. Diagnosis of Rheumatic Fever Reappraisal of the Jones Criteria: The Indian Experience The New Zealand Medical Journal. Vol. 10, p. 391, June 1988, part-II. No. 847.
10. Padmavati S, Prevention of Rheumatic Fever. Rheumatology Seapel 1988, Experta Medica. pp. 26–28, 1990.
11. Padmavati S. Rheumatic Heart Disease: Prevalence & Preventive measures in the Indian Sub-continent. Heart Aug/2001 86 (2), p. 127.
12. Padmavati S. Rheumatic Heart Disease in the SAARC Countries past present & feature direction. Quarterly Journal of Cardiology. Jan. 2002, 7(1), pp. 1A–3A.
13. Padmavati S, Bhatia Durge. Control of Rheumatic Fever/Rheumatic Heart Disease in India Through School Health Services. Executive Summary of an ICMR Pilot Project. ICMR and AIHF (Published in 8/2002).
14. Padmavati S, Acute Rheumatic Fever & Chronic RHD. A4 Century Review & Special Reference to India 2011 (JP Bros Med. Publisher), pp. 31–34.
15. Padmavati S. RF & RHD. Cardiology Text Book by M Khalilullah & SK Sharma 2012, Chapter 25, pp. 397–401.

Hypertension

1. Padmavati S. Kasliwal RR. Epidemiology of Hypertension in Indians & Approaches to its Control. Tropical Cardiology. Vol. XIII (Supp.) 1987, p. 19.
2. Development of methodology for prevention & Control of Hypertension in Developing Countries. WHO- CVD/88.5, 1988.

3. Self Measurement of Blood Pressure. Bulletin of the WHO. 66 (2), pp. 155–159, 1988.
4. Weight Control in the management of Hypertension Bulletin of the World Health Organisation. 67 (3), pp. 245–252 (1989).
5. Physical Exercise in the management of hypertension. Journal of Hypertension 1991, 9, pp. 283–287.
6. Alcohol & Hypertension: Implication for management Bulletin of the WHO 69 (4), 1991, pp. 77–382.
7. Can Non-Pharmacological interventions reduce doses of drugs needed for the treatment of hypertension? Bulletin of the World Health Organisation 70 (6): pp. 685–690, 1992.
8. Padmavati S. Specifications of a Control Programme in a Developing Country (India).Report of the Fourteenth Conference of the WHL Council Held on May 6, 1992 in Berlin, Germany, August 1992, pp. 13–17.
9. Strassee T. Relative costs of Artihypertesnive Drug Treatment Journal of Human Hypertension (1992) 6, pp. 489–494.
10. Padmavati S. Assessing Hypertension Control &Management WHO Regional Publications Europeans Series No. 47, 1993. Preliminary Results from India, pp. 173–181.
11. Padmavati S. Prevention of Target Organ Damage. Journal of Human Hypertension (1996) 10, Supp. 1, pp. 585–587.
12. Teaching the Teacher: A WHO/WHL Cross Cultural Project for Training Health Personal in menthods of patient education for hypertension CVD prevention 2 (1), March 1999.

Ischemic Heart Disease & Epidemiology

1. Padmavati S, Epidemiology of Cardiovascular Disease in India Ischemic Heart disease Circualtion Vol. XXV, April 1962, pp. 711–717.
2. Padmavati S, Gupte S, Pantulu GVA. Dietry Fat Serum Cholrestrol Levels & Incidence of Atherosclerosis in Delhi Circulation XIX (6), June 1959, pp. 849–855.

3. Padmavati S. The Cardiac Patient in Underdeveloped Countries American Heart Journal 58 (3), pp. 418–424, September 1959.
4. Bjorck Gunnar, Chavez Ignacio, Myasnikov Alexander L, Okeke Nlogha E., Padmavati S., Shillingford John P., White Dudley Paul. World Report on the Heart & Circulatory Diseases. The AHA, pp. 1–16, 28 November, 1962.
5. Padmavati S., Krishneswamy Kamla, Ghafoorunissa. Coronory Heart Disease. Nutrition in Major Metabolic Disease Edited by C. Gopalan, Kamla Krishnaswamy 1997, pp. 110–126.
6. Padmavati S. Epidemiology of Coronary Artery Disease in India. In Gopalan and Shetty (eds.), Diet, Nutrition and Chronic Disease: An Asian Perspective, Smith-Gordon Nishimure, 1998.
7. Padmavati S, Gupte Usha, Aggarwal HK, Chronic Infection & Coronary Artery Focus on Chlamydia Pneumonia. IJMR 2012, pp. 228–32.

Preventive Cardiology

1. Padmavati S, Kasliwal RR, Dhar A, Modi S, Arora AP, Gujral V, Omar A. Epidemiology of Coronary Heart Disease in India- A Long Term Prospective Study. Proceedings of International Congress of Preventive Cardiology, Moscow 24–27, June 1985.
2. Padmavati S. Preventive Cardiology an Introduction (Edited by HS Wazir) "Epilogue" Preventive Cardiology for India.
3. Padmavati S. Preventive Cardiology. CSI Souvenir 2012.
4. Celebrating the first 10 years of Nature Reviews Cardiology. Nature Reviews Vol. 11 Nov. 2014.
5. Top 10 cardiovascular therapies and interventions for the next decade, Valentin Fuster.
6. Celebrating the first 10 years of Nature Reviews Cardiology. 2014 and other articles- Dec. 2014
7. Decade in Review—Peripheral Vascular Disease: 10 years of breakthroughs in peripheral vascular disease. Mark A. Creager.

8. Decade in Review—Valvular Disease: Current perspectives on treatment of valvular heart disease. Friedrich W. Mohr.
9. Decade in Review—Cardiomyopathies: Cardiomyopathy on the move. Magdi H. Yacoub.
10. Decade in Review—Heart Failure: 10 years of progress in HF research—what have we learned? Henry Krum.
11. Decade in Review—Hypertension: The past decade in hypertension—facts, hopes and hypes. Thomas Unger.

Miscellaneous

1. Padmavati S. Editorial Special Cardiovascualr Problem in India. Indian Heart Journal, Vol. 17, No. 4. October 1955.
2. Padmavati S. 40 years of Cardiology in India. Souvenir CSI November 1988.
3. Padmavati S. Cardiology in Delhi: A trip down memory lane. XIV Annual Conference Souvenir, September 5–6, 1998, pp. 9–10.
4. Padmavati S. Kargil & The Simla Summit XV Annual Conference of Cardiological Society of India Delhi Branch Souvenir 4–5 September 1999, p. 15.
5. Padmavati S. The Many faces of Tobacco in India. Keynote address at Watch, 2000.
6. Padmavati S. Development of India's Healthcare Services. An update. 2001 year Book Marketing Cooperation with Southern and & East African Countries. Published by Institute of Marketing & Management.
7. Padmavati S. Cardiology in the 21st Century and the Indian Perspective. The Indian Journal of Chest Diseases Allied Sciences 44 (4), October-December 2002.
8. Padmavati S. Development of CVTS Surgery in India. Indian Journal of Thoracic & Cardiovascular Surgery. 20 (1) (Supp.) Jan/March 2004.

9. Padmavati S. 50 years of the Asian pacific Society of Cardiology in Retrospect: Long-Term Perspective. Indian Heart Journal November/December 2005, 57 (6), pp. 778–779.
10. Padmavati S. Manpower Requirements for Cardiology & Cardiac Surgery in the 21st Century. Cardiology Today 15 (4), July-Aug 2011, pp. 146–48.

Chapter 4: Professional Life

The All India Heart Foundation Golden Jubilee of 1962–2012. The International Society & Federation of Cardiology its components historical data 1950–1990. Mario R.Garcia Palmieri.

The International Society of Cardiology (ISC) and CVD Epidemiology. University of Minnesota School of Public Health.

http://www.epi.umn.edu/cvdepi/essay/the-international-society-of-cardiology-isc-and-cvd-epidemiology/

Chapter 5: Offshoots of Professional Life

Dr. Paul White

1. Paul Dudley White. My Life and Medicine: An Autobiographical Memoir. Gambit, 1971.
2. Paul Dudley White and Menard M. Gertler. Coronary Heart Disease: A 25-year Study in Retrospect. Medical Economics Co. Book Division, 1971.
3. Oglesby Paul. Take Heart: The Life and Prescription for Living of Dr. Paul Dudley White. Harvard University Press, 1986.
4. Paul Dudley White and Helen Donovan. Hearts: Their Long Follow-Up. W. B. Saunders, 1967.

Dr. Helen Taussig

1. Helen Taussig. Congenital Malformations of the Heart, Volumes I-II. Harvard University Press, 1960.

Dr. Ancel Keys

1. Ancel Keys. The Benevolent Bean. Farrar, Straus and Giroux, 1972.
2. Ancel Keys. How to Eat Well and Stay Well: The Mediterranean Way. Doubleday, 1979.
3. Ancel Keys. Adventures of a Medical Scientist: Sixty Years of Research in Thirteen Countries. Crown Printing, 1999.

Chapter 6: Historical Data and Ancient Systems of Medicine

1. Peter Pormann. Discovering Medicine in the Golden Age of Islam. Commentary (Royal College of Physicians, London), August 2013.
2. WHO Traditional Medicine Strategy 2002–2005.
3. Farkhunda Jabin. A Guiding Tool in Unani Tibb for Maintenance and Preservation of Health: A Review Study. African Journal of Traditional, Complementary, and Alternative Medicines.
4. AYUSH Government of India. 2010. Retrieved from http://indianmedicine.nic.in/index3.asp?sslid=133&subsublinkid=14&lang=1on 7 April 2010 at 17:15 IST.

    Wikipedia, author? 2011. Humorism. Retrieved on 7 April 2011 at 17.00 IST.

www.ingramcontent.com/pod-product-compliance
Lightning Source LLC
Chambersburg PA
CBHW030807180526
45163CB00003B/1183